PRAISE FOR CANCER WARRIORS

"*Cancer Warriors* reminds me of how frightening the cancer journey is even when the outcome is successful as in Bonnie's case. As physicians we sometimes forget the fear and anxiety people feel and how brave they are. We are so focused on the technical aspects of treatments. Thank you for writing this book; it reminds me to consider how people perceive what is happening which helps me be a better doctor. I hope it is inspirational to others going through this."

Dr. Rene Gonzalez
Professor of Medicine
University of Colorado School of Medicine

"Bonnie's honest and forthright style draws the reader into her journey through the pains, fears, frustrations, and hopes of dealing with cancer. Her honest and forthright style kept me glued to the pages and believing that God truly walks with us even through the worst of life's trials."

Roy Hanschke
Author, Speaker and Christian Radio Personality

"Bonnie Doran has so eloquently captured the array of emotions experienced through the cancer journey, but most importantly, she has captured the essence of hope! This common thread of hope is something I witnessed in all of my amazing cancer warriors and ends up being the very thread they often cling to during the darkest days of the journey. This devotional serves as a vital reminder of the power of hope for all those walking this difficult journey. Thank you for pouring your heart into this so that so many can be inspired!"

Sara Gause
PA-C, MS in oncology, founder of Awaken CARE

CANCER WARRIORS

52 DEVOTIONS FOR CANCER PATIENTS AND THOSE WHO LOVE THEM

CANCER WARRIORS

52 DEVOTIONS FOR CANCER PATIENTS AND THOSE WHO LOVE THEM

BONNIE DORAN

ILLUMIFY MEDIA GLOBAL
Littleton, Colorado

Published by
Illumify Media Global
www.IllumifyMedia.com
"Write. Publish. Market. *SELL!*"

Library of Congress Control Number: 2019920309

Paperback ISBN: 978-1-949021-88-2
eBook ISBN: 978-1-949021-89-9

Cover design by Debbie Lewis

Printed in the United States of America

To my husband,
who traveled this cancer road with me.

CONTENTS

ACKNOWLEDGMENTS

Writing doesn't happen in a vacuum. Here are some people who helped me in this process:

Megan DiMaria and Lynnette Horner, my critique partners, who gave me honest feedback and made the book better.

Michael Svoboda, my friend and coworker, who challenged me to write a devotional from my journals.

Karen Bouchard, Erin Grantham, Deb Hall, Mike Klassen, and Geoff Stone from Illumify Media Global, who guided me through the book publication and marketing process.

Debbie Lewis, for her awesome cover design.

Jennifer Clark, typesetter.

Numerous people, too many to mention, who encouraged me along the way.

STRANGER

BY BONNIE DORAN

Cancer was a stranger to me
Until I was diagnosed with malignant melanoma.
Joy was a stranger to me
As I struggled with the grief of a truncated life span.
God became a stranger to me
As I screamed, "Why?" and got no answer.
After four years of treatment,
Cancer became a constant but unwelcome companion.
Joy visited occasionally
With days of lessened fatigue, visits from friends, and sunny weather.
God never left.

INTRODUCTION

Why did I write this devotional book? Because I've been where you are. I've experienced the fear a cancer diagnosis instills, the side effects that seem worse than the cure, and the uncertain future.

In 2014 I had a mole gone bad. The surgeon dealt with it.

I thought I was done with cancer.

In 2015 the oncologist discovered a second melanoma. I underwent another, more painful surgery.

I thought I was done with cancer.

Since cancer could still linger on a microscopic level, in January 2016 I began a journey using immunotherapy. What followed were two months of side effects—vomiting, diarrhea, fatigue, rash, brain fog, and edema.

I didn't just think I was done—I felt done in.

Yes, I've been there. Throughout this journey, however, God has walked beside me. At times I couldn't feel him. At times I was so angry it surprised me he didn't leave me to my own devices. I've faced fear, anger, doubt, pain. You know what? God was still there.

I don't know what kind of cancer you face or what the doctor's prognosis is. I don't know what kind of treatment you'll receive or what side effects you'll suffer. Every cancer patient has a different pair of shoes and walks a different path.

I hope this devotional will encourage you. I hope you'll find comfort in knowing others have trodden similar trails. I pray that somehow my experiences will bolster you through the journey none of us want. I've been there, and so have others.

And God has been there. Above all else, I pray you'll cling to that truth.

A MOLE GONE BAD

Nothing can go wrong.

—Public address system to visitors in *Westworld*,
a movie in which androids run amok

I didn't think much about it at first. A mole on my left upper arm bled when I toweled off. I hadn't noticed it before.

My husband John noticed. "You should see the doctor."

"Sure." But I didn't want to. I'm not fond of going to the doctor. And what if it were nothing? I'd be so embarrassed.

Then my therapist noticed it. It seemed to have grown. "You should see the doctor."

"Okay, okay." I can take a hint.

One friend told me not to worry. She had basal cells removed all the time. The doc would just freeze it off, and that would be that.

The nurse practitioner looked at it. He numbed the area, scraped off the mole with a razor, and said he'd send it to a pathologist.

I didn't worry. Just a basal cell.

My first reaction to the procedure was relief the nurse could use a scalpel in the clinic then send the tissue to a pathologist. He didn't have to send me to a dermatologist or other professional, which would amplify my anxiety and, I thought, waste my time.

I didn't realize how much the process was affecting me until I was close to tears on the way home from lunch with friends. I'm sure part of my emotional upheaval was from getting numbed and having the mole scraped off. Most of my reaction was worry over whether they'd find a more serious cancer than a relatively mild basal cell or squamous cell carcinoma and if so, what kind. Up to that point, fear had hidden in my mind, but now I played those "What if?" games.

After a week of bone-crushing anxiety, a nurse from the clinic called. The mole was malignant melanoma.

I didn't know what a melanoma was. I only heard the word "malignant." Didn't that mean it was cancer and it had spread? Was a mole gone bad going to kill me?

I got that call while meeting my friend Megan for lunch. I was a mess. I'm thankful she prayed for me on the spot.

When I got home, I found additional messages. The nurse had set up a dermatology appointment, which included surgery. Surgery?

In the next message, the nurse told me the dermatologist wanted me to see a surgical oncologist right away. This was serious. She faxed all my info to a surgeon at St. Joseph Hospital in Denver, close to where I live. His scheduler would call me. Oh, and the doc would do biopsies on my lymph nodes. That sounded like *real* fun.

My husband rushed home as soon as I called him about all this. We called the "prayer Marines": his mother, my sister, and two writing friends. John also called his business partner.

At this point, we were all in shock.

Cancer? Me?

Lord, wherever we are in this cancer journey, fear snaps at our heels. Help us to trust you amid the chaos of appointments, surgery, and chemotherapy. Amen.

A LESSON FROM C. S. LEWIS

In grief nothing "stays put." One keeps on emerging from a phase, but it always recurs. Round and round. Everything repeats. Am I going in circles, or dare I hope I am on a spiral?

—C. S. Lewis, *A Grief Observed*

I have a sneaking suspicion the emotional journey through cancer all patients and caregivers experience is like what C. S. Lewis endured after his wife died from cancer. Lewis is a Christian author best known for his *Chronicles of Narnia* novels.

Like Lewis, we wait for something to happen. Will we be miraculously healed, suffer horrible side effects, or reach remission? Our life is on hold. Making plans for that cruise, working for that promotion, or knitting that afghan seems pointless.

Coming to terms with cancer is like dealing with grief. Depending on which model you prefer, grief has several stages.

The website Journey-Through-Grief.com lists seven:
1. Shock
2. Denial
3. Anger
4. Guilt
5. Sorrow and Depression
6. Acceptance
7. Engaging Life

The list comes close to what I've encountered. And like C. S. Lewis, I keep revisiting each stage.

Shock and denial hit me about the same time when I was first diagnosed. Malignant melanoma? No, that mole was just a basal cell. Invasive cancer happened to other people. I didn't quite deny the reality but tried to escape my diagnosis through television and other activities. I also referred to my cancer as "melanoma," because it seemed less threatening than the "C" word.

Reality hit. I cried a lot. Along with this came paralyzing fear. To me, cancer was a death sentence. My grandmother, uncle, brother, and brother-in-law had died of cancer. I knew what it could do.

Anger took center stage next. Friends had assured me the mole gone bad was a basal cell and the doc would remove with it a touch of his scalpel. I felt betrayed.

God got the brunt of my wailing and railing during that time. *How could you let this happen, God?* I knew as a Christian I wasn't immune to problems, but this felt like too much.

Guilt? I had survivor's guilt along with other guilts. My brother and brother-in-law were much younger than I when they died. Why was I going to live longer?

I also struggled with the certainty I could have prevented it. *Why hadn't I noticed it sooner? Why didn't I see the doctor when my husband suggested it? Why didn't I use heavy-duty sunscreen at the beach?* It was *my* fault I had cancer. Somehow, I had it in my head I was defective.

Sorrow weighted me as I thought of all the things I wish I had time to do. With a truncated life span, it wouldn't be possible. And I'd be leaving a grieving husband who deserved better.

Depression also hit. That's my natural tendency, but the feeling was amplified. I couldn't write. I couldn't face emails or anything on social media. I plodded through my daily routine like an old donkey unable to lift its hooves. *What's the point of it all? Should I just plan my funeral?*

Loneliness added to my mood. I didn't tell my friends. I didn't meet with other cancer patients. Every time someone asked how I was, the standard "I'm fine" came through clenched teeth. That squashed any comfort they might have offered.

Let's look at acceptance. Maybe I could climb out of this hole. I'd read *A Grief Observed* several years earlier, taken from Lewis's journal entries after the death of his wife. What struck me was his raw, uncensored grief as well as his gradual emotional and spiritual ascent.

Instead of burying my nose in science fiction and fantasy novels, I realized that my escape tactics didn't alter reality. What helped was reading the biblical accounts of Jehoshaphat, Hezekiah, and Nehemiah who overcame incredible obstacles with God's help. Could that same God help me?

Eventually I began to reengage in life. I adjusted to the new normal and took up the challenge of writing about my journey.

Yes, I have cancer. Yes, the outcome is uncertain. As I write this, I've been cancer free for a year. However, every CT scan I'll endure over the years will come with the "what if it's back?" agony. I cling to the hope my anguish will become faith and my uncertainty will become trust in God.

Join me in this process and plan for the future, even that cruise.

Lord, it's easy for us to get wrapped up in dealing with cancer. We forget that working through our emotional upheaval takes time. Thank you that you're always there regardless of our stage along the journey. Amen.

ACTION STEP:
Read *A Grief Observed* by C. S. Lewis.

MUSICAL CHAIRS

Plans are established by seeking advice; so if you wage war, obtain guidance.

—Proverbs 20:18

I got dizzy from the army of medical personnel I saw within a few short weeks.

For starters, a new registered nurse practitioner (RNP) for my primary care physician examined the mole. She had my regular RNP examine it before they scraped it off.

Another nurse (also from the doctor's office) called to inform me the mole was malignant melanoma. She scheduled an appointment with a dermatologist for a few days later who told her I should be sent to a surgical oncologist. The oncologist's scheduler would call me to set up an appointment. All those calls took place the same day. In musical chairs, it would have taken less than a minute before five chairs disappeared from the circle.

The scheduler called later that day. She'd set up an appointment with the surgeon for the following week. In the meantime, I exchanged Facebook messages with my sister-in-law, who suggested calling the

Mayo Clinic and researching the best hospitals. Maybe I should have gotten a second opinion as she insisted, but the thought of one more chair being pulled out was enough to discourage that idea.

And when my dentist's office called, I politely told the receptionist I would schedule my visit later, thank you very much. I told the same thing to my optometrist.

The game of musical chairs continued in the hospital as the medical professionals prepared me for surgery. I met with the nuclear medicine technician, the surgeon, the resident assistant, the anesthesiologist, and the surgery nurse. I felt like a slab of beef.

Whew. And that was just the *first* surgery.

I ping-ponged between assurance and head spinning. Were all these people exchanging information, or was it up to me to manage this? Hey, I was stressed enough. I didn't need to play musical chairs of who-has-what-record—records that included summaries of every visit plus CT scans, PET scans, MRI scans, and probably others I've blocked from my memory.

I would have done a lot better if I had remembered God was the ultimate surgeon, but by that time I was mad at him for allowing me to get cancer in the first place. All this rigmarole for one stupid mole seemed like—um—overkill.

Of course, none of this circus was a surprise to God. In the middle of all of it, he was the one constant. I wish I'd recognized that sooner, before I started wondering if my head was still attached after all the whiplash.

Lord, all these crazy appointments with all these crazy people can really fray our nerves. Help us, in the midst of it, to find your peace and perspective. Amen.

OPINIONS ARE LIKE BELLY BUTTONS— EVERYBODY HAS ONE

"Meaningless! Meaningless!" says the Teacher. "Utterly meaningless! Everything is meaningless." What do people gain from all their labors at which they toil under the sun?

—Ecclesiastes 1:2–3

One of the things I found frustrating in this cancer journey was the number of people eager to give me advice. They meant well, but I was skeptical of some suggestions.

A positive attitude I can understand, but a coffee enema?

Nice thoughts rely only on our own feeble power. Meditation can calm my nerves but can't remove the cancer from my body.

Regular exercise? That's important for everyone, and I don't get enough. My Fitbit obsessively reminds me I need to move. I'll accept that suggestion.

Eating right? Also important. However, eliminating every bit of sugar from my diet won't starve cancer because it always finds a way to steal sugar from other sources. And I found it difficult to accept the latest sure-cure food.

One book I read touted chiropractic care three times a week in its suggested cancer-fighting regimen. I failed to see how it would help.

Treatments and cures abound outside the medical field. There are plenty of treatments within medicine as well: surgery, chemotherapy, radiation, and immunotherapy among others. With medicine advancing so fast, it seems there's a new treatment announced every week.

Oh, I haven't mentioned *where* to get this treatment. An oncologist connected to a hospital? A special treatment center? A university hospital? And where will I have to go to get the treatment? In state, out of state, or out of the country?

We can drive ourselves crazy with all these questions. At best, we can find a treatment, alternative or not, that cures us. At worst, we can do or take something that doesn't work and delays treatment with something that would.

With all this hunting for the right treatment, we sometimes forget the real source of treatment: God.

God knows what will work. He made us and knows us individually. We must do our homework, but he will provide the right course of action, either through a doctor's referral, a friend's advice, or other resources.

We still might not like the outcome. After four years of treatments that included two surgeries, immunotherapy which caused horrible side effects, and a clinical trial, the doc found an immunotherapy drug that worked for me and that I tolerated. I don't like the fact that I took this drug for over a year before reaching remission. I'll still need CT scans to make sure the cancer doesn't return, an ever-present worry.

I thank God for leading me from my primary physician to a hospital oncologist to one of the best melanoma specialists in the world, located only twenty minutes away from my home—not counting rush hour.

We need to stop chasing our tails or the next big thing in treatment and rest in God's leading.

Martha opened her home to [Jesus and his disciples]. She had
a sister called Mary, who sat at the Lord's feet listening to
what he said. But Martha was distracted by all the
preparations that had to be made. She came to him and asked,
"Lord, don't you care that my sister has left me to do the work
by myself? Tell her to help me!"
"Martha, Martha," the Lord answered, "you are worried and
upset about many things, but few things are needed—or
indeed only one. Mary has chosen what is better, and it will
not be taken away from her."
—Luke 10:38–42

5

HOW COULD GOD DO THIS TO ME AGAIN?

"Have I not commanded you? Be strong and courageous. Do not be afraid; do not be discouraged, for the LORD *your God will be with you wherever you go."*

—Joshua 1:9

On October 7, 2015, I learned I had melanoma again.

I'd detected a lump on my arm near the original surgery site. I wanted to schedule an appointment with my surgeon, but he was booked for the next three weeks. I made an appointment anyway but also made a much earlier appointment with my dermatologist. Two days later, I learned the awful truth.

He performed a punch biopsy near the site of the original melanoma. He thought it might be scar tissue, but just to be sure . . .

He numbed the site. He put a lot of pressure on my arm in getting the instrument in place. It was deeper than he anticipated. He ended up with three good samples, and I ended up with three stitches.

As I waited for the biopsy results, my emotions bounced around like an unbalanced washing machine. The doc was probably right; it was only scar tissue. Even if it were another melanoma, I would just have another surgery to remove it. It couldn't be that serious. If the bump was nothing, I wasted all that worry. But of course, I panicked because I assumed it *was* something to worry about. I started wondering if my melanoma had metastasized into Stage V or worse and my days could be numbered in months, not years.

I ticked off possible outcomes:

- God flat-out heals me.
- The dermatologist got it all with the biopsy.
- He didn't get it all, and I'd have to have more surgery. I'd been down that road before.
- It metastasized, and I would have to go through chemo, radiation, and side effects.

My faith vanished, replaced by uncontrollable anger. It wasn't fair. I'd had enough of God's "tests" that supposedly would make me stronger. He wasn't answering my prayers or anyone else's. I was disgusted with my attitude, and I imagined God was too. If I were God, I would have drop-kicked me into the next universe.

The biopsy revealed another tumor. I immediately called the surgeon, certain he'd want to operate right away. I'd hoped our relationship was done, but here I was. No one returned my call.

My trust in God tanked even further. How could he let this happen again? I sat on the couch with a big glass of wine and a cat on my lap. Elspeth showed more sympathy than God.

And of course, the call from the dermatologist's office had happened while my husband, John, was piloting his private plane with a friend from out of town. When they got back, we'd have dinner together. I didn't want to see Steve. I didn't want to eat. I wanted time alone with my husband. In other words, I wanted to brood.

To top things off, we were leaving the next day for California to be with my sister and her family. My grandniece Gracie was having a fourteen-hour surgery to correct three different heart problems. She was thirteen days old! We were all focused on her.

But I felt neglected. I had cancer. No one seemed to care.

A nurse called the morning we left. The surgeon had reviewed the pathology report and would see me on the October 20 as originally scheduled. She told me to enjoy our vacation. If the doctor wasn't worried, I shouldn't be. Right? But I kept "boinging" on an emotional trampoline as my brain jumped among possible outcomes.

Friends assured me God was in control, even with this cancer. The platitude I heard so often, "God is good, all the time," rang hollow. I knew it was true, but it only added to my boiling rage.

I felt properly chastened when I read the day's devotional, which reminded me of God's promise never to leave me. I also half-remembered verses in the first chapter of Joshua about being strong and courageous. God helped me realize he would give me that strength and courage. He didn't expect me to (and he knew I couldn't) dredge up courage on my own. Still, I was a long way from claiming the promised land.

All this stress caused one of the worst arguments my husband and I have had in our thirty-six years of marriage. Of course, we forgave each other eventually.

In retrospect, I learned my anger hadn't ruined my relationship with God any more than my argument with my husband had ruined our marriage. If my hubby could love me through this strain, then God could as well. I gained a faith—at least for a little while—that couldn't be shaken.

Again the one who looked like a man touched me and gave me strength. "Do not be afraid, you who are highly esteemed," he said. "Peace! Be strong now; be strong."
—Daniel 10:18–19

ACTION STEP:
Practice deep breathing. Breathe in God's love and strength. Breathe out anger and fear.

6

OUT OF HER HANDS

My times are in your hands; deliver me from the hands of my enemies, from those who pursue me.

—Psalm 31:15

A writer friend of mine titled one of her novels *Out of Her Hands*. That's as true for me as it is for one of her characters. Healing is not under my control. It's a hard truth.

We like to pat ourselves on the back during therapy. We've chosen the right oncologist. We're eating (when we can eat) foods that nourish us. We exercise when we can. And we do other things to cure ourselves of cancer. We've got this.

No, we don't.

We love to think we're in control, but cancer never cooperates. It doesn't always respond to treatment. We could be treated with a drug that has to be stopped because of side effects, one that doesn't affect the tumors at all, or surgery that doesn't remove everything.

We don't want to lose our hair, but our hair has a mind of its own.

So does our stomach when we vomit everything up. Oh well. It didn't taste good anyway.

Another illusion is we can push God into doing things our way. He'll answer our prayers for healing if we pray long enough and hard enough. He may heal us but not because of our praying with a special formula.

I prayed a long time, as you and your loved one have, for healing from cancer. When I was first diagnosed, I ranted at God that he couldn't do this to me. I was his child, right? When the cancer recurred, I really lost my cool. *How dare you, God!*

What's hard to grasp is the fact that I'm not in control. God is.

I don't have any answers, pat or otherwise, for what we go through as patients or as caregivers. I believe, however, that God is in control, not us.

We can't see past the next doctor's appointment, CT scan, or infusion. And we can't see the end results. God can. God has a plan that goes beyond treatment.

As I posted in my Facebook group about my treatment progress, a friend suggested I turn those posts into a devotional book. I fought that. It was too personal. I'd written bunches of devotional pieces (sixty-seven to be exact) but didn't want to do a book. I wanted to write sci-fi novels. At the time of my cancer, one novel was published, another was finished, and I was working on a sequel. I was *not* going to write a devotional book.

Then my literary agent called. He'd been unable to sell my second novel, and we parted ways. Suddenly that novel wasn't my focus. Nothing was.

In the middle of all my ranting about having cancer, God promised I'd be a blessing to others. I couldn't figure that out at first, but then it hit me: what better way to help/bless others than to write a devotional book about my experience? In retrospect, that's why I'd written all those devotional pieces in the past (honing my skills) and why my friend kept bugging me.

With God's help, I started writing the thing I'd sworn I wouldn't write. I wouldn't have thought of this, but God did. His plan went far beyond my cancer.

God has a plan for each of us beyond our struggles. I don't know how God will use cancer in your life, but he will.

He's got this.

Lord, we think we're in control, but we're not. Help us to let go of our illusions and trust you. Amen.

7

PLEASE DON'T SAY THAT

It is an easy thing for one whose foot is on the outside of calamity to give advice and to rebuke the sufferer.

—Aeschylus

During my time of uncontrolled vomiting and diarrhea, my husband held my hands one night across the dining table. "Promise me you won't give up." His words said more about his worry for me than about my imminent demise. No one except my husband could have said this.

My therapist thought I was going to die, and she didn't see me at my worst. She wisely didn't bring it up at the time. She told me two years later, and it shook me even then.

So please, don't tell me I'm going to die.

Don't tell me a cousin's first husband died of the same cancer or so-and-so's cancer came back. Tell me instead President Carter received the same drug and is now cancer free. I can figure out I might not have the same success, but then again, I just might.

Don't insist some other doctor or treatment would be better than what I have. I received such a suggestion. That person should have done a little research. My hospital is one of the best in the nation, and my oncologist is one of the top melanoma specialists in the world. Why should I go traipsing around the country when the best medical help was twenty minutes away?

Reminding me I've had a good life isn't helpful when I feel I'll soon be robbed of half of it.

Please don't tell me of the miracle cures you discovered through the internet. I was fighting for my life. Telling me to eat more blueberries because of their antioxidants wouldn't make much difference, but cancer-tailored drugs might. And did, even without the blueberries.

Even hospital staff doesn't always get it right. I called a social worker who pressured me to take a walk. That would have been great advice to get me moving and make me feel better if I'd been capable of it. I couldn't do more than stagger down the driveway.

Some of the things I dreaded hearing were only in my imagination, and I'm glad they stayed there. *You look terrible. Have you put your affairs in order? Are you sure you don't need hospice?* Don't say it unless you know me very, very well. I don't take kindly to people who suggest what to write on my tombstone.

Here are some things you *should* say and do:

- Tell me how to counteract the edema that has swelled my legs into unappetizing, fat sausages.
- Give me the recipe for your egg drop soup or ginger tea.
- Tell me about foods I could probably tolerate, like yams.
- Do offer to sit with me during treatment or to provide transportation when my hubby is unavailable.
- Do ask me what I can tolerate before bringing over your famous lasagna.
- Tell me it's okay if I take a nap in the morning *and* the afternoon.
- Assure me of your concern. Ask me how I am. A hug is always welcome, unless you're squeezing the surgery site.

- Tell me you're praying for me.

And if you're in doubt about what to say, don't say it.

> **Gracious words are a honeycomb, sweet to the soul and
> healing to the bones.**
> **—Proverbs 16:24**

8

I'M RADIOACTIVE

I praise you because I am fearfully and wonderfully made; your works are wonderful, I know that full well.

—Psalm 139:14

Who knew a simple surgery could turn me radioactive?

The surgeon explained that in order to find the lymph nodes he wanted to remove I would need to be injected with a radioactive dye. That didn't sound like much fun to me, but the procedure fascinated my electrical engineer husband.

When we first arrived at the surgery waiting area, we were escorted to Nuclear Medicine. The technician told the nurse it was too early to inject me. The radioactive dye had a short half-life, which meant it would decay to half its strength in only a couple hours. The stuff had to be put in my system just before surgery so the doc could see the lymph nodes.

The tech escorted me to surgical pre-op, where the nurses set up my IV and put those compression thingies—excuse me, *pneumatic compression devices*—on my legs. When the time was right, they unplugged everything and wheeled me back to Nuclear Medicine.

The tech first injected me with a numbing agent, then shot the mole area four times with the radioactive dye so he could get all sides. We waited a half hour before he could take pictures of the lymphatic system and another half hour so he could take more pictures. He finally mapped the nodes under my arm by marking my skin with a black Sharpie pen. Nothing like the combination of high and low tech to give you confidence.

In the meantime, John and the tech had a wonderful conversation about the dye. What was it? Where was it manufactured? What was the half-life? At least someone was having fun—at my expense!

A year later I had a PET scan to check for cancer which again required a radioactive tracer. After the outpatient procedure, John couldn't wait to get me home and use his Geiger counter. The instrument's needle swung to its maximum reading. I'd pegged the instrument from three feet away. After he went back to work, he asked me to log the measurements every half hour as the radioactivity decreased.

What amazes me isn't the radioactivity so much as the complexity of the human body. The lymphatic system, among other tasks, delivers antibodies to the areas that need them. The surgeon had to remove lymph nodes from the melanoma site because the lymphatic system is too efficient. Any cancer the antibodies can't kill could be distributed throughout the body.

The immunotherapy drugs I received were intended to boost the immune system so the body could take up the fight against this virulent invader. In fact, when one tumor I could feel on my upper back grew even bigger, the oncologist assured me that was how it was supposed to work. The antibodies had rushed to the scene.

No one in their right mind would want cancer. It shouldn't be there. But I'm grateful modern medicine can work *with* my body to help it in the fight.

Lord, thank you for the body you've given me, but it doesn't always function the way you intended. Please give oncologists and researchers the wisdom and guidance they need to create more effective means to eliminate the cancers that shouldn't be there in the first place. Amen.

9

HOW NOT TO CELEBRATE THANKSGIVING

An hour of pain is as long as a day of pleasure.

—English Proverb

I misunderstood the nurse when she explained the procedure for my second surgery. She said I'd be under sedation, which I assumed would be a trip to la-la land while still conscious. I learned just before surgery that I would be completely out.

I wish I'd known that. Usually I get nauseous with anesthesia. I would have asked the nurse if she could give me something to ease that. Instead, after the surgery, I went through the whole vomiting thing until the next morning.

I cautiously ate a light breakfast and had no unwelcome results. Yay! But could I go to a Thanksgiving potluck and not be tossing my cookies every so often? I hated the idea of not only missing a good meal with friends but also disappointing my husband.

With some worry, we went. John said we'd "make an appearance." Instead, we stayed late. I should have known.

When we arrived, I enjoyed a small glass of wine but skipped the appetizers. I *started* to go easy on Thanksgiving dinner but couldn't resist a taste of every offering: turkey, dressing, mashed potatoes, and curry (one of the guests was Indian). I hoped for the best.

My tummy cooperated. We enjoyed hanging out with these wonderful friends. Unfortunately, I'd forgotten one important thing: my pain meds.

As the evening progressed, my arm started throbbing. And throbbing. Soon I scanned my arm to see if someone had put it in a vise. I hinted more and more insistently for John to take me home. "Hinted" is the right word. I wasn't clear that I really, *really* wanted to leave.

Then someone brought out a Scrabble game. I love Scrabble; so did everyone else. I had to wait my turn to play until someone went home and gave up their spot. I wish I'd known then about the Scrabble apps available on cell phones. I could have enjoyed my fix without causing myself serious trouble.

I played, although my throbbing arm distracted me from doing my best. Soon, the vise tightened as if I were in a torture chamber.

We went home. I made a beeline for meds and bed. Because I'd let the pain go so long, it took a while to get it under control. The common wisdom is to keep ahead of the pain. Obviously, I didn't listen to wisdom, pain, or plain old common sense.

I hadn't been realistic in gauging the surgery's effects. I should have known better. I'd been down this road before.

In retrospect, I should have scheduled the surgery for another time. Duh. I could have resolved the nausea with drugs before or even after surgery. I could have taken my pain meds with me to the party or begged John to grab them from home. Shoulda, woulda, coulda.

Don't let yourself or your loved one suffer the same consequences. Listen to your body before it starts screaming.

Lord, it's easy for us to get so wrapped up in our activities we forget to take care of ourselves. Help us remember that before we regret it. Amen.

THE SCAR

Search me, God, and know my heart; test me and know my anxious thoughts.
See if there is any offensive way in me, and lead me in the way everlasting.

—Psalm 139:23–24

After my first surgery, I had a scar. I didn't know what to do with it.

Since the surgery was performed on my upper arm, everyone could see the gash if I wore short sleeves. I didn't know whether I wanted to hide the scar or show it off.

The doctor removed flesh the size of half a golf ball so he could get clear margins around the melanoma. Since the incision was round, he couldn't just sew it up like that. So I ended up with stitches on either side of the hole, twenty-two total. On top of that, my arm now had a depression from that substantial chunk taken out. It was a beauty to behold.

Therein hung my dilemma. Part of me wanted to hide the scar with long sleeves after the nurse removed the stitches, hoping no one hugged me on that side. The other part was to go for the sympathy angle and all the attention it brought. "Oh, you poor dear . . ."

I tried both approaches with limited success. People *did* hug me on that side. Ouch. I didn't gain much sympathy because most people wouldn't look at it, maybe afraid of saying anything to hurt my feelings.

That was 2014. The scar was even worse when the doc performed another surgery a year later, the day before Thanksgiving, and cut out a portion four inches long, two inches wide, and up to an inch deep. Now I really had something to show. During that long Thanksgiving day—before the surgery site started to throb and before I begged my husband to take me home—I did receive the sympathy I was hoping for about my scar.

This scar thing is a metaphor for the emotional scars we all have. We can sport relatively small ones and expose them to close friends. We might elicit "You poor dear" or maybe some advice that is the emotional equivalent of a cream to make the scar fade in time.

Meanwhile, we don't show anybody the giant, painful scars that refuse to fade. They're too ugly.

We can try to hide them, but nothing is hidden from God. He's not shocked or uncomfortable by them. Instead of sympathy, God offers comfort, a lessening of the pain, and real emotional and mental healing, even if we've built up big, fat callouses around them.

It's hard to expose those deep scars. It's hard and scary. But we can trust God to heal.

**Lord, only you know the deep wounds we carry. Search us,
know us, and lead us to wholeness for your name's sake.
Amen.**

HOLDING THE LADDER

Kick away the ladder and one's feet are left dangling.

—Malay Proverb

One cold Saturday, I steadied a sixteen-foot ladder as my husband installed LED lights in his airplane hangar.

I'm glad I did, because it kept the ladder from wobbling. I was there to call 911 if the unthinkable happened and he fell onto the concrete floor. I could also break his fall, although having a 230-pound-hunk of a man flatten me wasn't my idea of fun.

My hands froze from gripping the cold aluminum rungs. He stepped on said hands, for which he apologized profusely.

I took other risks in holding that ladder as well. For example, while my hubby detached the defective fixtures and wired in the new ones, debris rained down. Fortunately, the fixtures themselves didn't fall on my noggin.

The operation was a success. My hands finally thawed on the way home.

Cancer treatment is a lot like climbing a wobbly ladder. Sixteen feet is a lot of climbing, especially when you're afraid of heights. When I'm smart, I ask someone to be my ladder holder. She can talk me out of my acrophobia.

My friends run a lot of risks. They bear the brunt of my complaints and anger with the situation. I'm sometimes thoughtless of their feelings or schedules. There's always the danger my depression or self-pity will flatten them. Sometimes loved ones can help. Sometimes they can't, and it's painful for them to watch me struggle to my feet.

I'm grateful for the ladder holders in my life. Who are your ladder holders?

He reached down from on high and took hold of me; he drew me out of deep waters.
—Psalm 18:16

BLOATED

"You blind guides! You strain out a gnat but swallow a camel."

—Matthew 23:24

One of my ongoing problems after stopping treatment with ipili-mumab was edema. I didn't even know what the word meant.

Okay, so my ankles were swollen. That didn't seem so bad.

My nurse recommended compression socks up to my thighs, but either I bought the wrong size or my legs were too swollen. John had to tug the things on for me every morning, which was a real chore. We finally gave up. At least I could ice my feet and put a pillow under-neath while I watched TV. That wasn't enough. My friend Jill insisted I needed to elevate my legs above my heart, even at night.

Then I couldn't wedge my feet into sandals or even slippers. Hospital socks became my closest friends.

My watches became a little tight until they didn't fit at all. Okay, so the edema was also affecting my arms. So what?

We finally went to the emergency room for other ongoing symp-toms, but edema wasn't on that list of worries. However, while there I could barely push my jeans over my hips the many times the medical staff asked me to disrobe. I reasoned I must have gained some weight. Right. How could that have happened with what little food I was eating that refused to stay in my stomach?

When I got home, I scoured clothing magazines for stretchy pants.

Fortunately, the doctors had a solution: an increased dose of levothyroxine for increased hypothyroidism. I started shrinking. Soon I could wear slippers. Then I could wear my loosest watch. Those stretchy pants threatened to slide right over my rear.

When finally got clearance to drive, my Weight Watchers meeting was one of my first destinations. I'd lost fifteen pounds, which was kind of nice because it immediately put me within my goal weight. A week later I was down another five pounds, which was due to the edema lessening. If "a pint's a pound the world around," I had carried at least an extra twenty pints of liquid and probably more.

The jeans that had been so tight were now baggy. I gleefully shopped for clothes a size smaller and was still amazed.

Much later, I discovered a spiritual lesson here. I had become so bloated in my life with all kinds of extracurricular activities that I'd lost sight of what was truly important.

A devotion by Kim Ramsey in *The Upper Room* devotional magazine rings true: "I was confusing busyness with holiness, wants with needs, and personal pride with ministry."

It's easy for us to rush from one appointment to another in our daily lives and forget to ask God what he wants us to do.

We need to cut back to the things that really matter so we can fit into the jeans of companionship God longs to have with us.

Lord, sometimes we get so busy we lose sight of you. Help us to cut out the bloat. Amen.

13

SCRATCH WHERE IT ITCHES

The itch is a mean, unconfessable [sic], ridiculous malady; one can pity someone who is suffering.

—André Gide, *Journals*, March 18, 1931

I love rashes, don't you?

A rash developing on the body signals an allergic reaction. Rash halted my first immunotherapy after just two infusions. As my oncologist started me on a different immunotherapy drug, I held my breath the little bit of rash I developed wouldn't progress to covering twenty percent of my body, or again the doc would have to stop treatment and come up with some other drug.

The rash with the first drug covered my whole body and became so acute the itching woke me in the night. The itching on my back had me constantly searching for a back scratcher (husband included) or the sharp corner of a wall.

My dermatologist took one look at my red, bumpy skin and prescribed triamcinolone acetonide—try to say that three times fast—a cream that worked wonders. Hubby applied it twice a day for weeks.

It wasn't a matter of my slathering it all over. I was so weak I couldn't lift my limbs, so he did all the legwork (pun intended) to get my calves within range. He was sweet enough to do my back, too, but I didn't like the cold shock of application. Couldn't he have warmed up the stuff?

The routine continued for a month, with John applying the cream in the morning before he left for work and in the evening before he tucked me into bed. The cream got smeared all over the bed sheets, but I was too tired to change them.

All of this taught me, among other things, my hubby loves me. I'm sure he would have liked to get to work on time or to bed on time, but he kept it up as we used jar after jar.

Another thing I learned was to be grateful for a dermatologist who prescribed the right thing and kept renewing that prescription.

I'm also grateful in a way for the rash itself. It signaled the doctors I was having an allergic reaction. If they hadn't stopped treatment, I could have been even sicker than I became. I can't imagine having more horrible side effects than those I suffered.

God sends spiritual rashes our way to change our behavior. Sometimes I go blundering through life without God's guidance, even when the choice I want to make seems a good one. I registered for a one-day writer's conference, then admitted I had way too much going on, like cancer treatments. Duh.

If I pay attention, I can see the warning signs and halt in my tracks before things get worse. I'd like to say I've learned my lesson, but I can be stubborn.

When I stop, even if I've messed up big-time, God can comfort me in the same way the cream eased my maddening itch. It doesn't happen overnight. But the best plan is to ask God's guidance in the first place.

Whether you turn to the right or to the left, your ears will hear a voice behind you, saying, "This is the way; walk in it."
—Isaiah 30:21

14

HAS ANYONE SEEN MY BRAIN?

A mind is a terrible thing to waste.

—Created as the slogan for the United Negro College Fund, 1972

My first cancer drug really messed with my brain.

I was so far gone I wasn't aware of it, but I should have guessed. I couldn't write. I couldn't even face the computer. When I finally could think coherently, I'd amassed thirteen hundred emails.

Stuck at home with way too much free time, I read the entire Harry Potter series but didn't retain any of it.

Because of brain fog, I couldn't drive per my doctor's orders. Even a short trip to the local espresso shop was outside my reach.

At one point I was convinced I had bedbugs crawling up my pant leg. John came home in a panic, thinking I did have bedbugs and we would have to fumigate the place. He figured out I'd been staring at the lint on my pants so long my eyes had played tricks on me.

I couldn't watch television. My world had shrunk to four walls, so world news seemed a foreign language. Instead, I took up people watching through our picture windows. People often jogged by or walked their dogs. Occasionally a nun from a nearby church joined the parade. I kept track of who drove what in our neighborhood.

Of course, I also watched for my husband's car. He was often working overtime and made daily trips to the supermarket before he came home. As soon as he walked in the door, I demanded service. When my edema eased and I finally could wear a watch, I discovered I was yelling at him every five minutes.

One day I noticed my elderly neighbor Alice across the street struggling while climbing up the stairs to her porch. She was lifting two thirty-five-pound bags of dog food for her Rottweiler and had to stop on every step to set down the bags. I tottered over but realized I couldn't help her. Two people strolling along the sidewalk hoisted the dog food to the porch stoop. I staggered home for more people watching. My husband was mad when he found out because I easily could have fallen.

Then there was the time I called 911.

Alice had stopped her car in the middle of the street and was talking with a young guy wearing a hoodie whom I didn't recognize. She kept her car door between them. I thought he was threatening her. I called the police.

When the two of them hugged, I realized they were friends and later discovered he was another neighbor.

Well, I called 911 back and said it was all right. They still had to send out a patrol car. How embarrassing.

When the officer arrived, Hoodie Guy talked with him. I went outside to assure the cop everything was fine. He probably thought I was some crazy woman spying on the neighborhood, which of course I was. The officer gave me a nonemergency number to call next time. I had the presence of mind to enter the number into my cell phone. Hopefully there won't be a next time. I later spoke with my neighbor (Adam) who knew Alice well and kept an eye out for her. My misunderstanding could have caused permanent damage. Maybe it has. I haven't talked to Adam since.

I could have used brain fog as an excuse that time. Looking back, maybe I should have instead of being so embarrassed. If you've had such an experience while suffering from chemo brain, give yourself some grace. Everyone will understand.

But so often when I have my mind firing on all cylinders, I say something before thinking. I seem to have a knack for hurting others by some thoughtless word. I'm fortunate to have small feet. I can jam them into my mouth more easily.

God gave us a good rule of thumb for weighing our words. We have two ears but only one mouth. In the future, I hope I keep that proportion in mind.

We all stumble in many ways. Anyone who is never at fault in what they say is perfect, able to keep their whole body in check.
—James 3:2

EAT! YOU'RE MUCH TOO THIN

Like newborn babies, crave pure spiritual milk, so that by it you may grow up in your salvation, now that you have tasted that the Lord is good.

—1 Peter 2:2–3

One of my challenges with side effects was keeping what I ate down or in. The treatment also affected my taste buds, so few foods appealed to me.

A sweet friend came over with peppermint tea and homemade soup. She also made a smoothie for me. Unfortunately, I hadn't screwed the blender onto the base tightly enough. The contents pooled on the counter and dripped to the floor. The kitchen ate well that day.

A couple writing buddies came over with lunch. I tried to do justice to the yummy spread, but my tummy wouldn't cooperate.

One of them returned a few days later with her homemade chicken broth, made me egg drop soup, and sat until I ate it all.

My sister-in-law suggested sweet potato. Facebook friends encouraged me to eat applesauce and yogurt. Good choices.

I received an anonymous mystery package with a box of tea and other goodies. And I managed to make a ginger tea with real ginger and honey from a recipe in the nutrition section of my cancer treatment tome. I couldn't handle much else in the kitchen with my lack of concentration.

Yogurt, applesauce, sweet potato, and soup. Not exactly a balanced diet, but at this point, unbalanced was an improvement from my constant vomiting.

Because of chemo brain, I couldn't drive to the store. Hubby made daily trips to the supermarket in a futile effort to find something I could eat.

I wouldn't have suffered so much had I taken the anti-nausea pills the oncologist prescribed. Alas, I either forgot (chemo brain) or they wouldn't stay down. Choking on pills one morning made me afraid to take any medication.

When I ended up in the emergency room because of my drastic weight loss, I stayed for an hour in an observation room while the doc determined if the steroids she gave me were effective and hadn't made things worse. While in the room, I discovered the hospital's closed-circuit TV. I could order breakfast online! I was hungry after nine hours at the hospital. So I ordered toast, eggs, fruit, coffee, and I forget what else. I also forgot what little food I could manage. I nibbled on toast, ate a bite or two of eggs, and contemplated the starving kids in Africa.

The fact is, without food to fuel my body, I'd become weak. It happens to me in a spiritual sense when I don't get enough Bible calories. In the physical realm, starvation is obvious. Spiritual malnutrition is harder to spot but no harder to treat.

Surrounding ourselves with supportive Christian friends is one ingredient of wholesome nourishment. Avoiding things that shouldn't be ingested—like pepperoni pizza or too-racy novels—is another ingredient. We also need to feed on God's Word and his presence.

Fuel up.

How sweet are your words to my taste, sweeter than honey to
my mouth! I gain understanding from your precepts; therefore
I hate every wrong path.
—Psalm 119:103–104

16

BRINGING HOME THE BACON AND THE CHEETOS

If you formed the habit of checking on every new diet that comes along, you will find that, mercifully, they all blur together, leaving you with only one definite piece of information: french-fried potatoes are out.

—Jean Kerry, "Aunt Jean's Marshmallow Fudge Diet," *Please Don't Eat the Daisies*, 1957

John and I were clueless at first about what, if anything, I could eat when food left my stomach one way or the other. He tried to find stuff that was appealing so he could fatten me up. It usually didn't work.

John doesn't cook. He solved the "what's for dinner?" problem by stopping at a supermarket after work every night to pick up something tasty.

Tasty would have been great, but my stomach and my taste buds couldn't agree on anything. Of course, I couldn't expect him to adhere to my diet of yogurt, sweet potato, and soup. I did my best to sample what he ate. But cinnamon rolls and bacon? It shouldn't have been on the menu. Pepperoni pizza? Ditto. And although Cheetos are one of my husband's favorite snacks, they certainly aren't mine.

Since my stomach wasn't cooperating, hubby resorted to other ploys: Gatorade and Ensure. I began to loathe the lemon-lime flavor. Ensure was okay until he insisted I finish the whole bottle every day before bed.

A lot of food succumbed to the "ugh" factor because treatment had weirded up my taste buds. Why eat if I didn't enjoy it when it went down and really didn't enjoy it when it came back up?

As I improved, my stomach settled but wasn't up to full capacity. When I was well enough to stagger out of the car, John drove us to a bagel place once. He insisted I eat more than one quarter of my bagel, but that was all I could manage. It was the same for anything I prepared at home, now that I could prepare simple meals.

Other things I find unpalatable at times are God's commands. How am I supposed to swallow "Love your neighbor as yourself" when she doesn't clean up after her dog? How can I love my enemy when he cuts me off on the freeway during rush-hour traffic?

Besides that quiet voice that exposed my bad attitude, I got embarrassing input from other sources. One billboard read, "Traffic is frustrating enough. Let someone in." I shouldn't have needed that reminder.

As we feast on God's Word, our actions become more in line with his desires. We need to absorb his love so we can pass it on to others.

Do not repay anyone evil for evil. Be careful to do what is right in the eyes of everyone. If it is possible, as far as it depends on you, live at peace with everyone.
—Romans 12:17–18

17

PARTY HARDLY

Pride goes before destruction, a haughty spirit before a fall.

—Proverbs 16:18

I'd planned a special party for my husband's sixtieth birthday on February 14, 2016. I invited a boatload of friends and gathered my favorite recipes.

Unfortunately, my body wasn't going to have it. My side effects had kicked in. We had to cancel. John told everyone I wasn't feeling well. Vomiting and diarrhea certainly qualified for that little excuse.

I postponed the festivities until March 13. This time I vowed I'd hold the party regardless of how I felt. It was potluck, so theoretically I wouldn't have much to do—just sit and look pretty. I hadn't had the energy to make anything—a disappointment for someone who loves to cook—but I knew people would bring more than enough food, and John planned to grill hamburgers. He still didn't think it was such a good idea. He was right.

As the party progressed and my energy disappeared, it was

obvious to my friend Melva I wasn't up to my hostess duties. She took over. What a wonderful gift.

Around 8:00 p.m., early as parties go, I needed to go to bed. John and Melva helped me up the two flights of stairs, then Melva got me undressed.

Unfortunately, our bedroom has no privacy. Any sound from downstairs gets amplified as it rises to the third floor, so it was unrealistic I would get some rest. The bedroom has no lock because it has no door, except for the one that leads onto the deck.

Melva became protective as one guest climbed the stairs to talk with me and another tried to come in from the deck. Thankfully, I was under the covers by then. Neither of them were aware of the situation, but Melva wanted to kick them down the stairs.

That party was memorable for everyone there but for the wrong reason: they saw how sick I'd become. The next evening, John took me to the emergency room. I didn't protest. The underlying problem (low thyroid) was easily treated, and from that point on, I improved daily. If only I'd waited another month to have the party.

Although it was gratifying to hear people tell me, "You look great," as I recovered in strength and weight, I knew the reason they noticed. They'd seen me at my absolute worst.

I can sort of laugh about the ridiculousness of that day, but I wish I hadn't let pride and misplaced determination take over. They propelled me into a social setting I was ill equipped for. I knew John and our friends would understand the situation. I didn't have anything to prove—except to myself. I wasn't that sick. I could handle it. Right.

Cancer treatment is not the time for us to deny reality or tough out an event we really shouldn't be doing. God and our friends will understand if we choose rest.

The anxiety we have for the figure we cut, for our personage, is constantly cropping out. We are showing off and are often more concerned with making a display than with living.
—André Gide

18

THE EMERGENCY ROOM

"And when you put this horn to your lips and blow it, then, wherever you are, I think help of some kind will come to you."

—Father Christmas to Susan, *The Lion, the Witch, and the Wardrobe*
by C. S. Lewis

As I continued to decline with lack of appetite, weight loss, and weakness, John insisted on taking me to the emergency room.

He'd wanted to take me weeks earlier, but I'd resisted. I wasn't that sick. My mother had been admitted to the hospital twice a year like clockwork because of bipolar disease. John had landed in the hospital with a blood clot and later in ICU with double pneumonia. No thanks. Emergency equaled hospital stay equaled a scary place to be.

Finally, after needing two people to help me climb stairs the night before, I relented. John told me, "If you fall, I can't pick you up." It was 9:00 p.m. on a Monday night.

Word to the wise: the ER is not where you want to be on a Monday night. We waited seven hours before I got any kind of attention.

Apparently victims of knifings and life-threatening illnesses got top priority. Mondays were the worst.

During this time, I texted some friends and read prayers from my mother's prayer book. Those prayers were all I could manage.

Finally I saw a nurse who took a lot of blood samples and hooked me up to a saline solution. I tried to give her a urine sample, but I was so dehydrated she needed to use a catheter.

The doctor finally came. She listened to my symptoms and squeezed my edema-swollen ankles. Her diagnosis? All my symptoms were consistent with low thyroid levels.

What? All my suffering could be traced to an easily treatable cause?

The doc ordered an injection of steroids, which would reveal whether this was indeed the problem. I felt better immediately but was moved to an observation room for an hour. After that, I was wheeled out of the hospital.

During this time, I'd been on my cell phone constantly with several friends, who came to the hospital and prayed for me. After they left, I texted them progress reports. I also updated my pastor, two critique partners, and my sister in California. Finally I had to sign off because I was losing battery power.

So what did I learn?

First, I learned to take my husband seriously when he suggests something, even when I'm not keen about it. I could have saved weeks of decline if I'd consented to go to the ER earlier.

Second, I learned to ask for support. Why hadn't I contacted my friends before? Like in *The Lion, the Witch, and the Wardrobe*, I would have had help sooner if I had called out.

And I learned God can meet me in the hospital, even when my prayer is as articulate as a trumpet blast.

Lord, help me to call for help. Amen.

19

SOCK IT TO ME

"So do not fear, for I am with you; do not be dismayed, for I am your God. I will strengthen you and help you; I will uphold you with my righteous right hand."

—Isaiah 41:10

At last I had a diagnosis. At last I had some hope I could be treated successfully. So simple: my symptoms were all consistent with low thyroid levels. All I needed to do was to go to my primary care provider and get an increased dose of thyroid meds.

Well, it wasn't so simple. John had his own doctor's appointment he couldn't miss. He wouldn't budge. My annoyance reached dangerous levels. Thankfully, God worked it out so the two appointments didn't conflict.

John had to drive me because I still couldn't wedge my feet into shoes. He helped me put on two pairs of hospital socks and get into the car.

Did I mention it was snowing?

He let me off at the doors into the clinic. I waited for him to walk me in, since I was still unsteady on my feet. We met with the doctor, got the prescription, and walked out.

John went to fetch the car and asked me to wait. The only thing that was warm was my hot temper. How dare my husband abandon me!

We finally got home. John helped me peel off the snow-soaked socks and put on warmer (and drier) slipper socks. He returned to work. I sank onto the couch.

I improved daily. Within a week's time, I could dress myself and turn over in bed. The edema diminished enough I could wear sandals and even my watch. I couldn't see the gradual changes at first, but John insisted I was making progress. I finally "got it" when I realized I'd just walked downstairs without taking the steps one at a time.

So what did I learn through all of this?

First, I learned how much my husband loves me. He insisted on taking me to the ER and sat with me for hours. He took time off work to take me to appointments. At home, as I mentioned before, he helped me on the stairs. He also slathered me with anti-rash cream twice a day and plied me with Gatorade and Ensure. Okay, I wasn't too sure about the last one. What a guy.

In a strange way, I realized how much God loves me. I didn't like the embarrassment of staggering around in hospital socks. I also didn't like the long recovery period. But he didn't let the side effects continue to the point of irreversible damage. He prompted my husband to cart me off to the emergency room, friends to pray, and a doctor to realize the underlying cause of my problems. God literally saved my life.

I don't know why I needed to go through all of this. Maybe God wanted to show me he never deserts me even in the worst of times. Maybe he wanted me to rely more on friends, a lesson I was slow to learn. And maybe he wanted me to lean more on him.

I pray I won't be so hardheaded next time.

Lord, you've been so faithful to me, even at the lowest times of my life. Help me to lean on your promises. Amen.

20

THE HAIR THING

If a woman has long hair, it is her glory.

—1 Corinthians 11:15

I didn't notice it at first. A few extra strands floated into the sink. Situation normal.

As I washed my hair, more and more strands clung to my hands and did their best to clog the shower drain. A little weird, but I still didn't worry about it.

But it continued. And continued. Soon I noticed the shape of my skull.

"I'm losing my hair!" I wailed.

My husband, always the logical one, told me as far as side effects go, hair loss was tame. Good point, but I didn't like it. Other side effects from my trashed thyroid had diminished when I got on a higher dose of medication. I didn't expect hair loss at this late date.

I contemplated whether to show off my soon-to-be-bald head. A friend of mine does that. She lost all her hair suddenly, and it wasn't due to cancer treatments. She didn't bother to cover her head. In fact, although she kept telling the gal at the espresso shop she didn't have cancer, the woman always offered free coffee. Making lemonade out of lemons, I guess.

I couldn't go that far. The hair loss embarrassed me. Sporting my baldness would announce to the world I had cancer. I didn't want the pity. I'd kept the disease a secret from even most of my friends. Telling people I had cancer made it more real.

So I contemplated a way to disguise it in case I really did go bald. Turbans didn't suit me since they screamed "Cancer!" The treatment center offered free wigs. No thanks. A friend undergoing breast cancer treatment did the most wonderful things with head scarves, but I never mastered scarf tying, even in Girl Scouts. My best hope was to find a hat that looked good on me. Fortunately, I never had to go that far.

My hair stopped thinning. As soon as my edema-swollen feet could fit into sandals, I visited my hairdresser. He worked wonders to create a hairdo that gave what I had left a bit of volume.

My hair finally started to grow. It was curly! It looked better but still wasn't back to its normal thickness. Friends told me my hair looked fine, but I still thought it was thin. I wondered if it would ever grow back to its former glory. In case you're wondering, it did.

In retrospect, I realize I was stressing a lot over this hair thing despite feeling better, unlike some cancer patients who showed up for their blood draws in a wheelchair, slumped over and apparently in pain. Instead of my constant complaints, I should have thanked God for his mercy, even in letting me keep a little dignity in the midst of cancer.

Another thing I realized: I was worried about my looks. I could hide the weight loss, edema, and rash. A bald head was harder to disguise.

Jesus said that God numbers the hairs we have. Trusting him amid treatment side effects is hard, especially with the hair thing. So I took a deep breath, prayed, and let go of this awful pride over my appearance. Letting go of vanity is something we all need to do.

Lord, forgive me for being so wrapped up in my negative self-image that I miss your blessings. Help me to let go of my pride and accept the situation, which for some reason you've allowed. I wouldn't mind more hair either! Amen.

WHAT ARE SISTERS FOR?

A friend loves at all times, and a brother is born for a time of adversity.

—Proverbs 17:17

You would think that with all the side effects I was experiencing and all the loneliness I felt by being stuck at home away from my various activities, I would have welcomed a visit from my sister, Pattie. She suggested it. Instead of accepting her offer, I told her I'd be fine. Our mother had been in and out of the hospital when we were growing up, so I resisted any admission I was sick.

Talk about silly rationalizations. I needed the companionship, and I really needed help during the day. I kicked myself for months for not taking her up on her offer.

There were extenuating circumstances, I reasoned. The timing would probably pull Pattie away from our nephew's wedding, which could have resulted in a lot of hurt and angry feelings.

And oh yeah, there was that pride thing. I didn't need help. And that denial thing. I was *fine*. Right. Violent vomiting and diarrhea were normal.

I had a lot of people locally who would have been happy to help if I'd just asked. I nearly cried when my good friend Megan told me, "Your friends would do anything for you." I could have asked for help. I didn't.

I used the lame excuse with my sister that I'd rather she visit when I felt better. She bought it. It wasn't strictly a fib, because we had a great time together when I was pretty much recovered. Still, having a nurse catering to my every need would have been a good thing.

A few people helped without my asking. Lynnette and Megan came over and fixed tea for us. Another day, Megan made me egg drop soup and sat with me until I finished it, as I mentioned earlier.

Two friends offered to take me to appointments. Judy sat with me in the oncologist's office, asked questions, and took notes. Mike drove me to an appointment in Boulder, about forty minutes away. Good plan. I needed help walking into the doctor's office and had double vision on the drive home.

Although I appreciated all this help, I felt like I was taking advantage of them and hated to feel like an invalid.

I'd like to say I learned my lesson, but it's still hard for me to ask. Praise God I haven't been that sick since. Next time, if there is a next time, I'll be more proactive. And maybe, just maybe, I'll respond to other friends who need help, even if they're as stubborn as I was.

Lord, sometimes we get so prideful. We deny we need help or refuse it when offered. Yet that help reflects your care, which is far bigger than the concern of our most loyal friends. Help us to ask gratefully and receive the gifts you offer us through others. Amen.

2 2

GETTING STRONGER

The LORD upholds all who fall and lifts up all who are bowed down.

—Psalm 145:14

Once the doc prescribed an increased dose of medication to support my thyroid hormones, I improved daily, or so my husband said. I couldn't see it most of the time since the process took over a month.

As I got stronger, I didn't need John to hold my hands as I took the stairs one step at a time. Then I didn't need him walking in front of me when I walked down the stairs in case I fell. I had gained enough confidence that I could manage all the stairs by myself. My "aha" moment came when I walked down one flight and realized I hadn't paused on each riser. Wow! A small miracle. I felt like a kid who'd finally mastered tying her shoes.

I stopped yelling at John every few minutes to bring me something from upstairs while I lounged on the couch. I could get it myself, much to his relief.

At church, when I had been at my worst, John would pull up to the curb. Rod, one of the greeters, would help me out of the car and escort me to my seat like an honored guest at a wedding. Soon I didn't need his help. I even started standing during music worship.

Friends had been accompanying me to doctor's appointments as well, but soon that was unnecessary. I didn't need anyone to help me walk from the car to the office.

Oh, and I could cook again. The brain fog had lifted, so I trusted myself around the stove, and now I could stand for longer periods.

I started to walk around the house rather than sitting on my bum because I really was feeling better physically and emotionally. In fact, I got a little antsy and walked in the neighborhood, although I used a walking stick "just in case."

My improvement didn't alter the heaved-up sidewalk, however. I fell twice, much to my embarrassment, once when my sister and I were walking home from my favorite espresso shop. Dang sidewalk. I tore the knee out of my new cropped pants, but that only made them more fashionable.

The other time was when John and I trekked to our favorite Italian place. Again, I blamed the uneven sidewalk. That time, I had an audience, which of course magnified my embarrassment. I'm glad I managed to get upright without too much help from hubby.

Why did I feel so ashamed to ask for help? I wasn't being realistic about my condition. Stubbornness in asking for help when I really needed it was a dumb idea when so many friends welcomed the opportunity to serve.

That attitude can creep into my spiritual life as well. *I'm doing just fine, God, but thanks for the offer.* I need to have my heart examined. The Creator of the Universe, who knows me better than anyone else, offers to strengthen my weak faith and to help me when I fail or to keep me from falling. And believe me, without him I'd spend a lot of time in the dirt.

To him who is able to keep you from stumbling and to present

you before his glorious presence without fault and with great joy—to the only God our Savior be glory, majesty, power and authority, through Jesus Christ our Lord, before all ages, now and forevermore! Amen.

—Jude 24–25

23

NOT TONIGHT, DEAR

Each one of you also must love his wife as he loves himself, and the wife must respect her husband.

—Ephesians 5:33

When I was at my sickest over a two-month period, John and I had to deal with sexual desire. He's always ready. Me, not so much with those side effects.

I had difficulty with moving in the first place. Even turning in bed was an ordeal.

John asked me to wake him when I needed to use the bathroom at night. I'd fallen a couple times. He'd hold my hands and help me to the toilet and back to bed. And he had to place me on the toilet and lift me off it when I was done. That embarrassment did nothing for my sex drive.

Neither did his slathering me with anti-rash cream. With my whole body gooped up, intimacy got left by the side of the road—uh, bed.

Depression didn't help the situation either.

So, with weakness, slathering, and lack of interest, we didn't indulge for a while.

John had great patience. Our marriage survived the strain. Our relationship is not about sex. However, society places so much emphasis on sex, it became a more important issue than it should have. I worried our curtailed intimacy pattern didn't live up to the hype and somehow we were subnormal.

"Not tonight, dear," is something I say often in other circumstances. I suspect you and your loved one have too. Pizza? Again? Not tonight, dear. Watch another horror movie from the '50s? Not tonight, dear, unless popcorn and cuddling come with it. How about driving to that sushi place across town? Not tonight, dear, I should be writing.

During treatment we might say, "Not tonight, dear," more often than usual. The trick is to know what we can and can't handle. I hate to disappoint my husband (except maybe with the pizza). Many of us are people pleasers. But it's not a crime to say, "Not tonight, dear," when we're too exhausted to think straight.

It's also not a crime to express our own needs. "Tonight, dear, I need to go to bed early." "Dear, could we take a drive in the mountains? I feel stuck at home." "Please, dear, would you grill tonight so I don't have to make an elaborate meal?"

We may think we're being too needy, but usually our spouses are happy to help. And in less strenuous times, we can say "Yes, dear" more often. It's usually a lot more fun.

Lord, sometimes it's hard to know when we should say, "Not tonight, dear." Help us to be sensitive to the needs of those around us, including our own. Amen.

A GIRL'S GOTTA GET HER NAILS DONE

*Little things seem nothing, but they give peace, like those meadow flowers
which individually seem odorless but all together perfume the air.*

—George Bernanos

When I could finally drive again, the first thing I did was make an appointment with my nail technician.

Forget the fact we had guests coming over for a twelve-hour movie marathon. Forget the fact that the nail salon was several miles away by freeway, and it would be my first drive since the side effects had finally disappeared. I was going to get my nails done.

I'd tried weeks earlier to hitch a ride to the salon but realized I was being frivolous. I found a nail file and worked on my claws. Now I was ready for a professional job.

I'm sure I shocked Marie as I tottered into the salon. I'd lost twenty pounds the hard way and was losing my hair. However, she had been through breast cancer and a double mastectomy. She understood side effects.

My nerves got a little frayed driving back home after a month of brain fuzz, but my nails and I did fine.

When I arrived home around 1:30 p.m., the movie reels had been going for an hour and a half. I was still shaky from the drive and probably needed to eat. I helped myself to a sandwich with my newly lacquered fingers.

I watched a couple movies with our friends and tried to keep the popcorn popping. We had no lack of food but not a lot of organization as people plopped the food they'd brought on the counter or wherever there was room. I usually put the potluck offerings on the dining room table, but this time I did a lot of armchair directing, with limited success. John kept to a strict schedule, which meant that during every five-minute break between films, a feeding frenzy and rush for the bathrooms ensued.

After two movies I was bushed. I went to our upstairs bedroom (third floor) to read in bed and get away from the—ahem—bedlam. My friend Rhonda came up and visited for a half hour since I couldn't handle the masses and the chaos. And because every sound seems amplified in our house, no way was I going to stack up a few z's.

Eventually I felt like being a good hostess. (I was also hungry.) I grazed and made more popcorn but generally let the moviegoers fend for themselves.

Finally, around eight o'clock, I pooped out again. I staggered up the stairs and read in bed until hubby kicked everyone out. He made an executive decision that ten was the new midnight.

No one noticed my nails, but I did.

Yes, getting my nails done was frivolous. But I needed to do a little something fun for my self-esteem. I don't do that often enough, even outside of cancer treatment. If this is you, do something for yourself that doesn't involve an IV.

Next stop: hairdresser.

Self-love, my liege, is not so vile a sin as self-neglecting.
—Shakespeare, *Henry V*

YOU LOOK GREAT

Self-pity comes so naturally to all of us, that the most solid happiness can be shaken by the compassion of a fool.

—André Maurois, *Ariel*

Friends and strangers alike say, "You look great," when I tell them I have cancer. I feel uncertain how to respond, other than an insincere "Thank you."

Let's face it. My body doesn't live up to society's ideal of the perfect shape. I'm overweight and getting more overweight. I'm hardly the thinnest reed in the marsh.

If people saw me two years ago, I'd agree with them that I look great or at least so much better than I did. Vomiting and diarrhea resulted in rapid weight loss as well as diminished strength. Watching me climb stairs one agonizingly slow step at a time while pulling myself up by the handrail would have made them cringe.

But I think the main reason these people continue to say I look great is they expect a cancer patient to look gaunt, strained, and bald.

Guilt weighs me down because I don't look like many cancer patients. I don't even wear a scarf to hide baldness.

Some patients do look normal. I saw evidence of this at a hospital-sponsored writer's workshop for cancer patients and caregivers. I didn't suspect that the woman sitting next to me had Stage IV lung cancer or that the woman across from me had a brain tumor that gave her seizures. And I certainly couldn't guess another participant had been placed in palliative care. The doctors couldn't stop the disease's progression, and death was imminent. These people seemed as healthy as anyone else.

I vacillate between wanting someone to say, "You poor dear," and wanting to hide behind false cheer. If they don't know about it, they'll treat me like a normal person.

I need to be at peace with myself and with this disease. People intend to be kind when they say, "You look great." Too often I dismiss their compassion. I know I don't look great.

But even without the cancer, I have a problem with self-image. I can't accept the fact that people do think I look great. My husband says it too, but he's biased. I continue to attend Weight Watchers meetings.

But someone really does think I look great, and that's God. He made me. I don't live up to his perfect design, but that's my fault, not to mention a result of the fall.

He doesn't stop there. He's more concerned about my attitude, about my ability to accept this body without condemning myself. I don't understand his love, which has no regard for my self-image, and I'm all too aware I fall short of his ideals of love and self-sacrifice toward others. He loves me anyway.

Maybe, just maybe, he'll help me encourage other cancer patients by sincerely complimenting them on a different level: their determination to stay the course without self-pity. I'm trying to be that way.

Thank you, Lord, that in spite of myself you love me anyway.
Help me to use your love as a launch pad to support others.
Amen.

HOPE FOR RECOVERY

Hope that is seen is no hope at all. Who hopes for what they already have? But if we hope for what we do not yet have, we wait for it patiently.

—Romans 8:24–25

When we first met Dr. Gonzalez at the University of Colorado Hospital, he impressed us with his expertise and ability to explain matters.

My first question as we talked was kind of a hedge. What I really wanted to know was how long I had to live. Instead I asked, "What is your goal of treatment?"

"To cure you."

Really?

"Everything changed in 2011," he said, referring to the year the first immunotherapy drug was approved by the FDA. He displayed various charts and scans on his computer. He showed us a graph of survival rates for patients with melanoma before 2011 and after. Before that important year, patients could expect to live for six to nine months. Now the life expectancy is ten to twelve years.

I didn't like the term "survival rates," but that's another issue.

He showed us before-and-after CT scans of one patient who had taken an immunotherapy drug. At the beginning, his body was riddled with cancer. The tumors shrank until they disappeared altogether—in two weeks!

Hope surged in me like a welcome ocean wave on a hot day. I could be free of this curse in a few weeks.

Of course, the doctor couldn't guarantee that, and it hasn't worked out that way.

My electrical-engineering husband became so enamored with this download of information—charts, graphs, and scans, oh my—that he asked for a copy. Dr. Gonzalez asked, "Do you have a flash drive with you?"

"No."

"Bring one next time. The file is too big to email." Then he paused. "I think that was from the presentation I gave in Iceland."

Iceland? I didn't think *any* conference would be held in Iceland.

A nurse told me during one of my many blood draws, "We're one of the top research hospitals in the country. As a result, we attract the best doctors."

Much later, we learned that Dr. Gonzalez is one of the top melanoma specialists in the world.

Medicine can't predict how a patient will respond. I had too many side effects to continue with the drug my previous oncologist had prescribed. I reacted badly to a clinical trial that had to be stopped. The third drug resulted in only fatigue and a slight rash. The doc couldn't find a tumor in the last CT scan a year after treatment.

As accomplished as the oncologist was, he couldn't predict the drug's effectiveness or my ability to continue those infusions. But my faith rests in God, not medicine, as the ultimate healer. God chose not to heal me as dramatically as some. I could still die of this disease and much sooner than I'd like. Another kind of cancer could pop up at any time. Those possibilities will always dangle on a thin thread over my head. Doctors are fallible. God is not.

I still have hope, because I know the One who's really in charge. And I have hope in life after life.

There is surely a future hope for you, and your hope will not be cut off.
—Proverbs 23:18

THAT WILL COME IN HANDY

A gift in season is a double favor to the needy.

—Publilius Syrus

When my new oncologist first examined me, he found a large tumor near the surface of my back, just under my rib cage. "That will come in handy," he said.

At the time, I had no idea what he meant and didn't ask. I discovered later the tumor indeed came in handy.

Dr. Gonzalez could palpate it when I went to the clinic every three weeks. He didn't need a CT scan to monitor the progression of the disease because he could feel the tumor was shrinking.

Early in my treatment, the tumor got bigger. I panicked. "Not to worry," he said. "It's supposed to do that in the early stages." All those antibodies were rallying to the site and swelling it.

Oookay.

Because the tumor was near the skin surface, doctors could do biopsies without having to thread the needle around organs and such. Piercing organs probably wasn't a good idea.

The tumor continued to retreat. It became harder for him and me to find it. During one visit, I tried to point it out to the nurse practitioner. I had been feeling around my back without success. "There. It's right there."

"That's your rib."

The doc continued to monitor that tumor, although I had many smaller ones on my chest wall. Every three months he ordered a CT scan. He displayed the new and older scans side by side on the computer screen to show us the progression of treatment. On one scan, the radiologist drew an arrow to show where the tumor was. The next one showed no tumors, but the doc decided to continue treatment for another three months.

As scary as that tumor was as I continued to press on it daily, it was a blessing because the doctor could monitor my progress more easily. God has a habit of using what we consider awful in our lives for our good.

May you or your loved one rest in the assurance he will bring something good out of cancer. As an example, look at the life of Joseph in the book of Genesis. His brothers sold him into slavery, his owner's wife falsely accused him of attempted rape, and the one person who could have had him released from prison forgot to mention it to the authorities. Yet these circumstances resulted in the deliverance of both Egyptians and Israelites.

We can rarely see God's design when our nose is against the black fabric of our lives. God is still weaving the threads of our lives into a beautiful pattern.

"You intended to harm me, but God intended it for good to accomplish what is now being done, the saving of many lives."
—Genesis 50:20

Action Step:
Read Genesis 39:1–41:40.

2 8

LET THE BAKING BEGIN

One cannot manage too many affairs: like pumpkins in the water, one pops up while you try to hold down the other.

—Chinese Proverb

When I first met with Dr. Gonzalez, he wanted to learn whether the first cancer drug was still working. He prescribed a vacation from treatment for three months, then retesting. I felt like a kid released from school for summer break.

I went wild with cooking and especially baking. I'm still dealing with the aftermath.

I discovered the Food Network channel on television and became addicted, especially to *Chopped*.

My reading material ballooned as I subscribed to cooking magazines in wild abandon. I amassed a total of five to join the one I already had. Later I added a sixth to the mix as well as a cookbook to join the others on my shelves. I now use a computer program that allows me to find recipes with specific ingredients in my ever-expanding army of cookbooks.

I bought recommended kitchen equipment, most of which was useful.

Many dinner recipes didn't appeal to John and me, including a recent try at puttanesca that turned out too spicy and salty for us to eat. A ton of baking recipes ended up in the oven, however. I didn't want those yummy desserts staring me at the face, so hubby took them to work where they were devoured. The mistakes never made it to his office. John insisted I had a reputation to uphold.

When I returned to the doctor after three months, the tumors hadn't changed size. He set me up in a clinical trial. Vacation was over.

Although that craziness with cooking eventually diminished, I still enjoy trying new recipes. But I only have so much time. I can't cook it all. I'm learning to pick and choose.

I've discovered the same thing in my life, which came to light as I sat at home. I couldn't do anything on my previously overloaded schedule, so I finally realized I couldn't do everything. With all that time, I thought through which activities were truly important. When I recovered, I cut out two writer's meetings. I needed to stop meeting and get back to writing. I even slowed my dead run of cooking to a trot.

The forced halt to my activities restructured my time. *Get a clue, woman. You have cancer.* Treatment had to eclipse everything else. All those tests, infusions, and doctor's appointments took a toll on my physical and emotional energy, not to mention time at the hospital and the strain of rush-hour traffic.

We need to take another look at our lives. It's easy for the sake of busyness to neglect family, friends, and especially ourselves. When we fill our lives with minutiae, we have no time to reflect on what's truly important. We need to sort through our activities, pray for guidance, and shape those activities around what God wants, not what society demands.

What is the use of running when we are not on the right road?
—German Proverb

PATIENCE

You can't set a hen in one morning and have chicken salad for lunch.

—George Humphrey, *Time*, January 26, 1953

I don't know why the medical world calls sick people "patients." When I endured cancer treatment, patience was not one of my strongest attributes. It still isn't.

During my first visit with Dr. Gonzalez, he showed us CT scans of one of his patients. The first scan showed tumors spread throughout his body. The second scan two weeks later showed NO cancer.

That man's first oncologist had given him a chilling prognosis: he had nine days to live. That doctor referred him to my doctor, perhaps as a last-ditch effort.

With time so short, Dr. Gonzalez decided to treat him immediately without waiting for confirmation he had the right gene to make the drug effective. In this case, *impatience* was a virtue. I don't recommend it for most circumstances, however.

The man got worse. His wife panicked. "Not to worry," Dr. Gonzalez said. That was the normal progression of treatment.

That patient suddenly began to improve. Two weeks later, the cancer was gone.

I was positive this miracle drug would cure me within two weeks as well, and I could go on with my life. However, God had other plans than a quick fix. This did *not* sit well with me. The truth was, since everybody reacts differently and this new drug hadn't amassed decades of data, the doc couldn't predict how long it would take before the cancer disappeared, if it ever did. My patience was tried again and again with every CT scan that showed the tumors were still there—shrinking, yes, but not fast enough to suit me.

The tumors were shrinking, but of course I wanted them *gone*. I was impatient to be declared cancer free and be released from the endless cycle of treatment. When would this wheel spinning end?

You or your loved one may be experiencing the impatience of being a patient. We can make a choice. We can fume about the delay and complain to everyone in sight, or we can lean on God's assurance he's in control of the situation, and he'll give us the emotional and physical strength to endure it. In my life of remission, I wish I'd mastered that reliance; I would have been a lot happier, and so would those around me.

Let him that hath no power of patience retire within himself,
though even there he will have to put up with himself.
—Baltasar Gracián

30

SELF-CARE

"Come to me, all you who are weary and burdened, and I will give you rest. Take my yoke upon you and learn from me, for I am gentle and humble in heart, and you will find rest for your souls. For my yoke is easy and my burden is light."

—Matthew 11:28–30

Self-care is not a dirty word.

We hate to burden our loved ones with what we think are unreasonable demands, and we hate asking for help. However, sometimes we need to care for ourselves by letting someone else care for us.

I needed a lot of help when I was at my worst. As I mentioned before, John slathered me with anti-rash cream. Now, I couldn't blame myself for wanting him to do my back, since I couldn't reach it. But my legs? Forget the fact that I couldn't bend down for fear of falling over. I didn't want him waiting on me hand and foot. (Well, actually, it was kind of nice.) I understand now I should have just let him do it and thanked him rather than grousing about it. I needed to assess my condition realistically.

Fatigue was a biggie as I went through side effects. Toughing out the day with droopy eyes wasn't the best choice. Succumbing to the magnetic pull of my bed was. I felt I was accomplishing nothing, and of course I needed to accomplish *something*. Let me tell you: the old American work ethic doesn't apply to cancer patients. What I really needed to do was stop burdening myself with "ought tos," show myself some love, and let my head hit that pillow.

When the oncologist released me from treatment for three months to give my body time to rest, I did what I truly loved: baking. I also, as mentioned before, subscribed to four *additional* cooking magazines, ordered a cookbook, and became addicted to the Food Network's *Chopped.* Anything worth doing at all is worth doing right. That was self-care for me. For you or your loved one, self-care may be watching the dogs at a bark park on a sunny day (wearing plenty of sunscreen) or enjoying a latte at your favorite coffee shop.

One of my attempts at self-care backfired. Friends encouraged me to get a massage. I'd never had one before. A place downtown wasn't far from my home, so I went. I filled out a ton of paperwork about my health. When the masseuse read through the questionnaire and got to the word "cancer," she paused. I told her I had a tumor on my upper back. "Show me," she said. After she felt the golf ball under my skin, she refused to treat me. A friend later told me that pressing on the tumor during a massage could squeeze the cancer cells into my lymph system. No massage.

I found other ways to be kind to myself. After the doc cleared me to drive, I made a beeline to my nail technician and had her give me a bright spring color. That boost in self-image was followed shortly thereafter by a trip to my hairdresser. I hadn't had a haircut in two months. Or was it three? Instead of overgrown tresses, he found thinning hair and had to design a style that would disguise it as best he could. Having a new do worked wonders for my self-esteem.

Find a form of self-care that works for you. Don't let those voices in your head tell you that you should return to your old job now, fix lunches for five kiddos and hubby, or volunteer to help at the food drive. You're worth self-care.

"Come with me by yourselves to a quiet place and get some
rest."
—Mark 6:31

ACTION STEP:
Take a nap!

31

WHERE'S P. D. Q. BACH WHEN YOU NEED HIM?

For our light and momentary troubles are achieving for us an eternal glory that far outweighs them all.

—2 Corinthians 4:17

Peter Schickele, aka P. D. Q. Bach, is a twentieth-century composer, musician, author, and satirist. Among the more than one hundred of his works are such humorous favorites as "Concerto for Horn and Hardart," "Trio (sic) Sonata for Two Flutes, Tambourine, and Tuba," and "Echo Sonata for Two Unfriendly Groups of Instruments." One of his compositions uses kazoos.

I wish he'd compose a new piece, "Concerto for MRI versus Orchestra."

I enjoyed several of these nerve-wracking scans. I empathize with those who have experienced more of them because they certainly rattle *my* brain.

The preparation isn't so bad, although I'm not a fan of those so-called gowns. I'm also not a fan of the ear plugs the technician jams in my ears. But the "fun" part is the scan itself.

Before my first MRI, the tech offered a choice of music while the machine pounded the innards of my cranium. I will never listen to Rachmaninoff's "Piano Concerto No. 2" again.

The party begins when the machine powers up and . . .

CLANG

CLUNK CLUNK CLUNK

EEE-OOO

I sighed in relief when the process was over.

The Magnetic Resonance Imaging scanner is an amazing piece of equipment. It shows the doctors what's going on more definitively than an X-ray and without radiation. But I'd pay good money (like I'm not already) for something a bit quieter. My attitude toward the MRI machine is like how I feel toward God sometimes.

Okay, God, I admit I need patience, but do you have to run me through all these trials to get there? And what about this cancer? Why, oh why, did you do this to me?

When I was having such horrible side effects from the first treatment drug, all I could do was rail at God and scream, "Why?"

The short answer: I don't know.

The longer answer: my cancer has given me more empathy toward other cancer patients, because I've been there. And I can now write about my difficult experiences so that maybe others can be encouraged.

I don't know how long I'll have the pleasure of these exams now that I'm in remission, since melanoma likes to camp out in brains. My oncologist isn't so much of a sadist that he'd give me extra ones, would he?

I try to be grateful for these marvels of science. It's not easy.

Cancer is one of the biggest obstacles in anyone's life, but we deal with smaller ones as well: a teenage daughter we must discipline all too often, a freeway driver who learned his dubious driving skills from "Wrecks Are Us," or a stupid computer like mine that doesn't know how to spell.

I need a better attitude.

Lord, it's so frustrating when I face big and small issues in life. Help me to look beyond the process and trust you for the outcome. Amen.

COUNTING THE COST

"Suppose one of you wants to build a tower. Won't you first sit down and estimate the cost to see if you have money to complete it?"

—Luke 14:28

When my oncologist suggested I enter a clinical trial, I was excited. I could contribute to science and be cured, all at the same time.

I had no idea what I was getting into.

The study coordinator gave me scads of paperwork to fill out. I committed to take the drugs as prescribed and to submit to periodic tests. I agreed to allow my test results to be reviewed by researchers. In short, I signed away my life.

The fun began with a CT scan. I had a blood draw, doctor's appointment, and infusion the next day. The following week, an ophthalmologist examined me to establish a baseline, since the treatments could affect my eyesight.

I received a chart on which to record when I took two drugs by pill. I had to explain any missed dose. And I had to take that chart and the remaining pills to my doctor every visit.

Each doctor's visit involved an EKG, part of the myriad tests the trial required. That wasn't too bad, although I wasn't a fan of having all those electrodes stuck everywhere then ripped off.

Then there were the blood tests. Lots of them. One blood draw required twenty-two vials. I'm glad someone explained that each vial held only a tablespoon of fluid. Otherwise, I would have been worried I wouldn't have any blood left. It became increasingly difficult for the nurses to find a good vein to use, which made the process even more fun.

The trial also called for CT scans every three months. They required I drink a contrast fluid and wait an hour before the procedure. The study threw in a PET scan for good measure. For that, I got a radioactive tracer that took an hour to work through my system. And let's not forget the MRI scans of my brain, with the scanning machine's clunk-clunk-clunk rattling my cranium. All of this was on the hospital's schedule, not mine.

The docs took two biopsies. I was fortunate I had a large tumor just under the skin. It meant they didn't have to maneuver around various organs to get a sample. But of course, it meant undressing, wearing a gown, getting a twilight drug for surgery, and the requisite recovery time. My hubby had to pick me up, cutting into his work. I spent hours at the hospital.

I felt like a failure when I developed serious side effects and was kicked off the clinical trial team. The coordinator of the program had to tell me repeatedly it was not my fault. Of course it wasn't. My body had betrayed me.

I suppose the data they collected was useful. It wasn't useful to my oncologist, although he could detect the tumor was shrinking. Because of the nature of a double-blind trial, my identity remained hidden. No one, not even the researchers involved, could match a patient to a test. I was just a number in the system. Perhaps the worst part was that the records were sealed. No one, not even my own oncologist, had access to the info, so it never got into my charts.

Although I'm still pleased I participated, the process itself caused serious side effects: low sodium and elevated liver levels, nausea, diarrhea, fatigue, and weakness. Almost every week, I had to show up on the hospital doorstep with arm bared for a blood draw and/or an IV for scans. I learned to wear certain blouses that had loose sleeves.

I didn't know what I was getting into. In short, I didn't count the cost.

That's what I often do in ordinary issues of life. I sign up for a Bible study then find out how much homework I must add to an already overloaded schedule. I take a supervisory role at a conference bookstore and end up missing workshops. Or I commit to helping someone when my days are too packed for a breather.

None of these are wrong. Some are good ideas, but not all of them at once!

My lesson: count the cost before you commit. Oh yeah, and ask God about it. I'm sure he has some ideas.

Everything is worth what its purchaser will pay for it.
—Publilius Syrus

UNINTENDED CONSEQUENCES

Second thoughts are ever wiser.

—Euripides

As I mentioned earlier, although I dutifully followed the requirements of the clinical trial, I developed serious side effects.

I continuously battled fatigue. Once I took a two-hour nap in the morning.

Overall weakness was also an issue. On some days, I depended on John to walk me through the hospital. Sometimes he helped me to the bathroom at night.

And then there was nausea and diarrhea, inconvenient at best.

The doc monitored every aspect of my health. It concerned him when my sodium levels plummeted and liver levels skyrocketed.

He took me off the infusions (I'd had one of the third drugs in the trial) and adjusted my pill dosages, eliminating one and gradually increasing another, hoping my numbers would stabilize so I could continue treatment. However, when we returned to the original dosages, the sodium numbers dropped again to their dangerous levels.

The nurse practitioner ordered me to drink two liters of Gatorade a day, which I didn't do consistently. All that fiddling didn't help. My liver levels were nine times above normal and the sodium extremely low. The oncologist hospitalized me for two days.

I couldn't understand it. Why was low sodium such a big deal? Then I remembered reading about a female marathon runner who died after a race. She didn't replenish the salt she lost through sweat. Yikes.

So, I thought, the nurse would give me an IV of saline solution and she'd tell me to eat more salt, right? Wrong.

The answer to my problem was not to increase my salt intake. The nurse gave me an IV drip of saline, but it made no difference. Instead, the powers that be restricted my hydration. For those two days in the hospital, they didn't give me much. What was worse, they had to help me to the bathroom every time I needed to use it. Then I got to sit on the toilet and pee into a cup that collected and measured my urine. Lovely.

At one point, I decided to go to the bathroom without the nurse's help. I unscritched those pneumatic compression devices, the squeezers that prevent blood clots from forming in the legs and that make sleep difficult if not impossible. I swung my legs over the edge of the bed, stood—and set off every alarm in the place. The nurses rushed in, realized I hadn't fallen or anything, and lectured me. I didn't realize I was a fall risk. Really?

After two days of this, I got discharged. Did they give me salt pills? No. Instead, the nurse instructed me to limit my water intake to 600 ml a day. That was hardly enough to wash down pills and brush my teeth.

I was a good girl. I poured water into a bottle with measure lines and kept that bottle with me. I went in every week for a blood draw. The numbers finally started rising. They increased my water limit and finally eliminated any restrictions.

My liver was another problem. The doctor prescribed prednisone. The dose was gradually reduced as my liver numbers gradually rose to within a healthy range.

The prednisone had unintended consequences. The drug can accelerate cataract growth. Within a year, both of my eyes needed surgery.

These side effects were unanticipated. Many times in life, our words can have unintended consequences as well. A thoughtless word can be misconstrued. One of my friends won't speak to me now because I disagreed with something she said. I posted a comment on Facebook and had to delete it because of the angry reactions I received. I also have made jokes that were inappropriate or hurtful.

We can't always take back the consequences, but we can avoid them if we think first, speak later.

The words of the reckless pierce like swords, but the tongue of the wise brings healing.
—Proverbs 12:18

34

TRYPANOPHOBIA

You will not fear the terror of night, nor the arrow that flies by day.

—Psalm 91:5

Trypanophobia, an irrational or excessive fear of needles, affects 3.5 to 10 percent of the population.

Needles don't bother me. What *does* bother me is the incessant poking, usually twice a day every three weeks when I would have a blood draw and an IV of my immunotherapy treatment. When I was fortunate enough to have MRI and CT scans, they required more pokes. Lots of fun.

I was the problem child. Because surgery on my left arm removed seven lymph nodes, nurses could only use the right arm. The major vein of my inside elbow (median basilic vein) was usually the target, but that vein got tired. The other veins played hide-and-seek. One time, it took two nurses and three punctures to find a vein that worked. Another time, the nurse wrapped my arm in a warm towel and used a vein visualization device that can detect veins under the skin. Fortunately, that procedure went smoothly and without hitting a nerve, which is another joy all by itself.

The clinical trial I entered in late 2016 used three drugs, one of which was administered by infusion (more pokes). The trial required an intense weekly ritual of blood draws (up to twenty-two samples at one time) and obsessive MRI and CT scans.

When something in that soup of drugs caused serious side effects, the doc threw me off the team. I started a different drug by infusion every three weeks in 2017. That drug was successful, but I was at it for over a year. I finally decided to get a port. In retrospect, I should have done this earlier and saved myself some grief and bruises.

A port-a-cath is a central line that is implanted under the skin. Its long, flexible catheter is usually placed in a large vein in the chest, with the business end (reservoir) just under the skin. It has three prongs that guide the nurse as she inserts a needle to draw blood or give infusions. Medical staff can use it multiple times the same day, and it's less painful than the usual method. It's less painful because I use a lidocaine cream to numb the area, covered by—get this—Press'n Seal plastic wrap. Hey, it works!

About twenty-five million patients get a peripheral venous line (needle poke) every year. For millions of cancer patients, getting skewered is a way of life. I'm not happy to be a part of that.

For me they're like the regular pricks to my conscience that God's Spirit sends my way. It's his way of telling me I need to change my behavior. Sometimes he has to do it several times to get my attention. When I respond, God does amazing things. He can extract my bad attitude like a blood draw and infuse me with his presence.

I need constant pokes from God to stop me from messing things up. Sometimes it hurts, but I'm grateful he cares enough to keep me on the right path and to give me the strength I need to follow him.

Lord, we don't like you to remind us of our shortcomings. Help us to respond in a positive way and to welcome the infusion of your love and teaching. Amen.

35

ANY OLD PORT

LORD my God, I take refuge in you; save and deliver me from all who pursue me, or they will tear me apart like a lion and rip me to pieces with no one to rescue me.

—Psalm 7:1–2

It was after a year of cancer treatments that I finally decided to have a port implanted.

Why did I resist for so long? My attitude was silly. Professionals and friends assured me it would ease blood draws and infusions. No more hunting for recalcitrant veins. No more tourniquets to make such veins more visible.

I read a lot about chemotherapy ports or port-a-caths, which can be accessed with less pain than needles. The surgery seemed routine and straightforward. However, when I saw one photo of a woman with a port that left a permanent, visible bump and scar, I freaked.

Why? Two reasons. That bump would brand me as a cancer patient, and it made this whole cancer thing more real.

Oh, and there was that whole surgery thing, which is not my idea of a good time.

I dreaded surgery day.

I'm so glad my friend Janet went with me to the hospital. She was a wonderful support. Besides, the hospital wouldn't let me have the procedure without someone there to drive me home.

We arrived early. I got to wear the usual gown. A nurse gave me what I hoped was the last puncture with a syringe. My head spun with the parade of nurses, residents, and others who traipsed through my pre-op room.

At last we were ready. Janet left me and the surgery nurse wheeled me into the operating room.

Once I was settled, the nurse placed the electrodes on various parts of my body. I got a blood pressure cuff that squeezed my biceps every few minutes. The nurse numbed the surgery site and draped a sheet over me that covered all but one breast.

I don't remember the surgery itself. The sedatives they use nowadays cause amnesia. I thought I'd enjoy watching the procedure despite my fears, but the nurses knew what they were doing by putting me out. They gave me some of the stuff ahead of time to calm me. The process was so routine that usually a physician's assistant got the job. I didn't care as long as the thing worked properly.

One friend quipped that using the port would be a great way to drink margaritas. I disagreed. What would be the point of *that*?

Recovery time in post-op was nil, but I staggered out of my room after the one-hour stay. I should have taken the nurse's suggestion and asked for a wheelchair. I'm glad I had a friend to lean on.

We grabbed lunch and a latte in the hospital cafeteria before the next procedure, a routine CT scan. After the port surgery, it seemed anticlimactic. The nurses left the IV in place so at least I didn't get poked twice. It made sense, but now that I had the port, I was disappointed they didn't use it.

One thing this experience taught me was that my fears, as usual, were unfounded. I couldn't remember the surgery, so I couldn't replay it in my mind. I had little pain afterward. The next time I had an infusion, the port worked like it was supposed to. And no one knew I had a port unless I showed them the bump under my skin above my right breast.

My fears were totally unfounded, but I couldn't escape them. I was relieved when the procedure was over, of course. My conversation with Janet as we caught up with each other's lives provided distraction that kept me from dealing with my reaction to the port and coming to terms with the fact that my cancer treatment was far from over.

I kept saying God had this under control. He did, but I fretted anyway. Many times in life, I let anxiety get to me instead of turning to God for his reassurance. It's tough to do that. I'm human. But God is still there if I make him my refuge when those fears come.

Maybe next time I'll trust God a bit more.

Lord, sometimes our fears threaten to eat us alive. Help us to trust you even amid a scary situation. Amen.

WHIPLASH

Hope deferred makes the heart sick, but a longing fulfilled is a tree of life.

—Proverbs 13:12

One day, I waited in the doctor's office while the nurse practitioner talked with the oncologist. She came back with the news that he wanted a PET scan instead of a CT. She also made an offhand comment that he didn't want to stop treatment. What?

Two months before, Dr. Gonzalez and I agreed that I would have three more months of treatment followed by a CT scan. Then we'd stop. I couldn't wait. No more trips in traffic to the hospital and back every three weeks. No more skewering me to access the port. No more three hours at the hospital for blood draw, doctor's appointment, and infusion.

The thought of three additional months of treatments when I was convinced I was nearly done threw me into a tailspin.

Also troubling was the doctor's change of mind on scans. Instead of a simple CT scan, he prescribed a PET scan, which is more precise at finding cancer cells. Did that mean he thought the cancer had spread?

Would it be like my previous experiences? I had surgery in 2014 to remove the first tumor. I thought that would be the end of it. Then another showed up in 2015. Did I still have cancer after battling tumors on my chest wall for two years?

While waiting for the PET scan results, I employed my favorite tactics to avoid thinking about my devastated hopes: reading, watching movies, and baking. They didn't change reality. Prayer didn't make me feel any better, but I should have remembered that emotions are fickle at best.

I posted on my Facebook group about this setback. The depression I expressed surprised even me. Was I really that upset? Well, yes.

A couple days later, I went to yoga practice. I tried to be nonchalant, but one yoga partner wasn't fooled. "Are you all right?" The tears forming in my eyes were answer enough. She prayed for me on the spot.

The following Sunday, she asked me again. Same tears. I hadn't slept well for several nights because of my tailspin, which didn't help. On top of that, my endocrinologist had reduced my thyroid medication. I heaped that on my worry pile as well.

After two weeks, I thought I was over the trauma. Judging by the amount of reading I did, maybe not. Some of that avoidance behavior was because I felt stuck in my writing, but not most of it.

I finally got back my balance and got back to my life—writing, laundry, etc.—but always with the worry about what that scan would discover.

When I finally got the PET scan, I waited anxiously for my doctor's appointment the next day.

We reviewed the scan together. No cancer and no more treatments! That day I had my last infusion. I even have a Certificate of Completion signed by the infusion nurses to prove it. And I rang the ship's bell on the way out to the applause of everyone in the infusion center.

My focus during this was all wrong. I concentrated on the worry instead of the God who had led me through this cancer journey for four years. I needed to trust him to orchestrate the length of treatment and its outcome. I might have had three more months of treatment.

The PET scan might have shown that my cancer had returned in full force. I'm grateful it didn't.

I don't know what will happen in the future. None of us do. But we know the One who's working in the midst of it.

In the time of trouble avert not thy face from hope.
—Hafiz

37

PATTERN WORK

Those who hope in the L ORD *will renew their strength. They will soar on wings like eagles.*

—Isaiah 40:31

As a private pilot, my husband flies in a pattern when he approaches an airfield. Often this means circling the airport either clockwise or counterclockwise at a specific distance and altitude before final approach and landing. Air traffic controllers give him instructions, which he repeats and follows.

When John initially contacts the tower, he tells them he is, say, ten miles out and requests either a "full stop" (he lands) or a "touch-and-go" (the plane's wheels touch the runway before he immediately takes off again). Occasionally he'll have to hold in the pattern until other traffic clears the area. It's not a good idea to land on top of someone else. Could get messy.

With any flight, there are checklists for preflight actions, run-up before flight, and postflight steps. The procedures are different for each type of plane.

When I was still undergoing treatment, I often felt like I was stuck in a flight pattern. Every three weeks I'd have a "touch-and-go" with blood draw, doctor's appointment, and infusion, only to repeat the process. The preflight and postflight actions of driving to the hospital and back added to my time. Unlike a flight, none of it was fun.

Flight planning also includes checking the fuel levels. We never run out of fuel, but many days I was flying on fumes with immunotherapy-induced fatigue.

Despite carefully monitoring the weather, John and I occasionally run into bumpy conditions. Those sudden downdrafts are especially scary. The air often smooths out, but sometimes the wind becomes too strong to continue safely. Similarly, in my cancer journey I experienced side effects a few times that made it unsafe for me to continue with the current treatment.

Cessnas and other planes require periodic maintenance after so many hours of flight time. So do I. For the next two years, I'll be under surveillance with CT scans every three months. I'll also have to get my port flushed with heparin every month to prevent blood clots until I have the thing removed.

I like to think of God as the pilot. I'm tempted to wrest control out of his hands (as if I could), but I'm glad he keeps the plane level. I've tried a couple times to take the yoke while John was flying so I'd be ready to handle the plane in an emergency. He'd say, "Let me take over," when I couldn't perform the simplest maneuver. What a relief.

I hated all the ups and downs of treatment, but now I can put the treatment plane in the hangar where it belongs. Although I enjoy flights in the Cessna, I hope my treatment plane stays grounded.

Lord, I feel like I'm still flying in circles after so many months of treatment. Help me to trust you to get me down safely. Amen.

CANCER GONE!

Praise be to the God and Father of our Lord Jesus Christ, the Father of compassion and the God of all comfort, who comforts us in all our troubles, so that we can comfort those in any trouble with the comfort we ourselves receive from God.

—2 Corinthians 1:3–4

I'd heard "we got it all" after each of my surgeries to remove melanoma. I was therefore skeptical when my current oncologist declared he couldn't find any tumors in the last CT scan.

The scans showed the size of my tumors was decreasing. In my previous scan, my largest tumor had shrunk so much the radiologist had to insert an arrow into the image to show us where it was. Still, I didn't expect this diagnosis. I figured I'd be having more treatments until—when?

The doctor gave me a choice in how to proceed at this juncture. One of his patients elected to continue treatment every three weeks, even though he'd told her the cancer was gone. She traveled from her home in Nebraska several hours away. I guess she was scared to death the cancer would return with a vengeance, as am I. And one patient, after stopping infusions, did have his cancer come back. He returned to treatment and again reached remission.

The doc's other comments bothered my husband. The doc said he didn't know when to stop treatment. The drug was so new it didn't have a track record. John didn't understand why he was being so cagey about it.

I decided to have another three months of infusions followed by another CT scan. The oncologist agreed. He wanted another CT scan before—what?

He never said, "cancer free," "in remission," or some other term. I learned later doctors are reluctant to use these words. For many patients, such a pronouncement is the gospel truth. Not so. Doctors are fallible. Disease progression is unpredictable.

Without the word "remission," we felt unsettled. Still, this was the first time no tumor had been detected. The doc was happy. Shouldn't we be?

To be honest, after such a long road of treatment, we were stunned. And unfortunately, we had no time to celebrate it. John went back to work and a looming deadline. I left directly from the hospital to a four-day writer's conference an hour away in the Colorado mountains. There I immersed myself in general sessions, workshops, and appointments with editors. John and I couldn't even talk over the phone because the conference location had no cell phone service.

Of course, I told everyone I knew about the news. Many had been praying for me, and they rejoiced with me, although it still seemed unreal.

I wondered where that left this devotional book on which I was still working. How could I speak to cancer patients still undergoing treatment when I was basking in sunlight on the opposite side? Wouldn't readers be annoyed?

Anyway, I continued writing, hoping the book would encourage and comfort others in the fight. That's what we're here for, right?

Comfort. That's one thing we can offer patients and their loved ones, whether it's a prayer, a hug, or chicken noodle soup. I urge you to be a comfort, regardless of your cancer path.

Lord, help us to encourage others in this journey. Amen.

3 9

DON'T WASTE YOUR CANCER

The quality of mercy is not strained;
It droppeth as the gentle rain from heaven
Upon the place beneath. It is twice blest;
It blesseth him that gives and him that takes:
'T is mightiest in the mightiest; it becomes
The throned monarch better than his crown.

—Shakespeare, *The Merchant of Venice*

Like talents, God gives us unique experiences while battling cancer. We can either hide them or use them to encourage others. Others suffer, too, and who knows? Maybe our conversation will be the balm they need.

When I got hit hard with side effects, I cried, "Why are you doing this to me, God?" Part of the answer, I believe, was writing this devotional.

Also, I could have been using this disease all along to encourage others. Sounds weird, doesn't it? Here are a few things I could have done:

Instead of hiding my cancer from most of my friends, I could have been open about it. The few I told felt privileged to pray for me.

Many welcomed the opportunity to serve. That blessed both of us. They came over with smoothies and egg drop soup. Friends on Facebook gave me advice on what I should eat. At that time, my tummy rejected every bit of food I sent down my gullet. But a sweet potato, my sister-in-law's suggestion, went down and stayed there.

I did a few things right. Once, John took me to the ER where we waited for seven hours. Those around me were in much worse shape than I, so I prayed for them. My brain was so scrambled that I couldn't express more than a help-and-heal kind of prayer, but God understood. And I had the presence of mind to ask several friends to come to the hospital to pray. They fell over themselves to work out their schedules to meet at my bedside. That blessed all of us.

If you're like me, you hate to have others help you. You think that it's weakness or that you're imposing. Neither is true. Swallowing my pride took a lot of courage. God turned it into a life lesson in realizing how much others cared.

Here's another situation: My husband John had a work deadline while I was too sick to leave the house. After a long day of overtime, he made daily trips to the supermarket for that night's dinner. I could have either asked someone to pick up a few groceries or asked the women's group at church to bring over meals, although honestly I had too much brain fuzz to think of it. Someone told me to have the store deliver them, but I don't remember—brain fog again—whether I suggested it to John or not. It certainly would have relieved him of some of the burden he carried.

I once took chicken soup to a friend after her hysterectomy and got blessed twice, first by cooking which is something I enjoy, then by having the opportunity to talk with my friend when I delivered it.

When I finally confessed my cancer woes to my neighbor, it opened a door in our relationship. We had a great conversation, something we rarely did with lives that seldom intersected. She offered to bring over dinner. While she set yummy stuff on the kitchen counter, I begged her from the bathroom to grab a few clean clothes for me upstairs because I—um—hadn't reached my destination in time.

Months later, I joined a writer's workshop for cancer patients sponsored by my hospital. My attitude at first was self-serving. I wanted the participants to help me with my devotional. Instead, we helped each other as we listened to prose and poetry about our struggles. Without sympathetic ears, these patients would have cried in the dark.

I'm still learning how to turn things around and not to waste my cancer. May you and your loved one join me in this journey of discovery.

Since you get more joy out of giving joy to others, you should put a good deal of thought into the happiness that you are able to give.
—Eleanor Roosevelt

40

REMEMBERING WHAT I WANT TO FORGET

Not the power to remember, but its very opposite, the power to forget, is a necessary condition for our existence.

—Sholem Asch

While writing this devotional, I was reminded again and again about my illness. I wish I could forget.

The original trauma was bad enough, but I relived it as I typed my previously handwritten journal entries. No wonder there were times I avoided writing.

I remember my first surgery, especially recovery. The first postsurgical nurse did nothing but stare at my vital signs. The second nurse engaged with me, but he was eager for me to pack up and leave. Apparently it was past the time the recovery room stayed open. He was kind enough to give me a vomit bag or two, which I utilized to the full on the drive home. It's funny the details that stick unbidden in my brain.

Oh, and I have a scar so I don't and can't forget.

I do have some things I want to remember, like one prompt and loving response when I reached out for help. As I shared in an earlier chapter, a friend told me, "Your friends will do anything for you." I want to keep that truth in my memory banks. I want to remember my husband's care and the prayers offered by so many.

But I want to forget the vomiting, diarrhea, and ten hours total in the emergency room. My brain fog during that time was a blessing because I can't remember some of those days.

My friend Carl remembered a potluck we hosted two years ago. "You were just lying on the couch." Somehow I carried on a conversation before my energy gave out and I needed to retire. I climbed the stairs with two people helping me and in full view of our guests. That was me at my worst. That potluck tops the list of things I want to forget.

In the same way, I can't forget regrets and downright sins in my life, even now that I'm healthy and have full control of my faculties. I've walked past someone in the supermarket who looked confused and needed help. I've said unkind words or failed to say a kind word. Everything gets tangled into a giant ball of guilt.

God has a selective memory, for which I am grateful. I don't understand how God can forget something completely, but he says he does. The Bible declares, "I, even I, am he who blots out your transgressions, for my own sake, and remembers your sins no more" (Isaiah 43:25). He is helping me to put this trauma and my sins behind me, although my brain will never forget them completely.

He doesn't remember my sins, but he does remember *me*. I sometimes wonder how I don't get lost in the crowd with seven (or is it eight?) billion people on the planet. But he does. And that's something worth remembering.

"Can a mother forget the baby at her breast and have no compassion on the child she has borne? Though she may forget, I will not forget you! See, I have engraved you on the palms of my hands."
—Isaiah 49:15–16

41

DON'T EAT! YOU'RE MUCH TOO FAT

"You are altogether beautiful, my darling; there is no flaw in you."

—Song of Songs 4:7

"You've lost another five pounds," the Weight Watchers assistant told me. That was five pounds lower than my goal weight.

The news thrilled me, though I didn't like the way I got there. I'd had uncontrollable vomiting and diarrhea for weeks. But I was more than ready to enjoy freedom from the scales.

I'd lost so much weight I could pull up my jeans without unzipping them. Even my underwear and bras didn't fit. I needed a new wardrobe. Oh, the suffering. I went on a serious shopping spree.

I still have those smaller clothes, but after eating to make up for lost pounds, I gained thirty-five. I'm not a happy camper.

Blaming my body is easy but not helpful. It's possible I went into starvation mode to conserve what fat I did have. When I started eating normally again, my metabolism didn't get the message I wasn't starving. That's what they say anyway.

But I went far beyond providing enough calories. Food tasted good again. I didn't have to worry about whether what I ate would stay down, so I ate pretty much anything I liked. That was fine to a point, but I needed to slow down and eat less. I didn't.

Exercise, or lack thereof, was another component. I'd become so weak I couldn't climb stairs or walk into a restaurant unaided. I hadn't even walked around the block in months. I couldn't manage yoga. I got lazy. And scared. The fear of falling hung over me. I did more lazing around than anything.

Eventually I returned to Weight Watchers and a determination to get myself back in shape. So far, it hasn't worked.

Yes, the weight's still there. The bulges won't budge. I'm convinced all my clothes shrank in the dryer. I moved those smaller clothes to another closet so they wouldn't stare me in the face. I bought two pairs of pants that fit my expanded waist. I only bought two pairs, thinking that would motivate me. Instead, I'm doing laundry more often.

That attitude leaked into my total self-image. If I couldn't control a simple thing like weight, how could I ever accomplish anything? That way of thinking became a merry-go-round of tree branches that slapped me in the face with every revolution.

My hubby doesn't listen to me when I wail about my weight. He says I look great. His biased vision reminds me God thinks I look great, inside and out. I don't understand it, but I need to accept it. It's true.

I'm working on changing my focus from the extra pounds to God's view of me. It's a hard thing. But if I see myself through God's eyes, I can walk tall instead of slouching.

Lord, it's ingrained in me to think of myself in rotten terms. Help me to change my focus and see myself through your eyes. Amen.

42

MOURNING THE LOSS

"I will turn their mourning into gladness; I will give them comfort and joy instead of sorrow."

—Jeremiah 31:13

While writing this book, I needed to refer to the journal entries I had written during treatment. I transcribed them into a Word document so I could easily find details.

When I reached the entries about side effects during my clinical trial, I wept. It took me a while to figure out why.

In reading through my entries, I discovered how sick I really had been. At the time, I was pretty much clueless. My journal laid out the details I'd conveniently forgotten.

While I was in the middle of everything, the effects didn't seem so bad. Seeing them described in my journal in one clump after another shook me.

I mourned.

Part of it was empathy for my past sick self who had gone through such horrible health issues. I had experienced side effects equivalent to those from drastic chemotherapy and radiation. Now, looking at things from the outside and knowing that several people thought I was going to die, I reacted with fear to that buried memory. It was the same fear I'd had at the time but had tucked into a corner while I was battling for my life.

In transcribing my journal, I learned I needed to separate myself from those experiences. Yes, it happened to me. Yes, it was life threatening. But I survived. I'm on the other side of that period in my life. It can't hurt me in the present.

I also mourn what I lost during that period. I lost time I could have used for writing. I lost hours at the hospital. With the first drug, I lost twenty pounds in about six weeks, which probably caused metabolism issues. Those issues are what I blame for my subsequent weight gain, although stress eating has also been a factor.

With the clinical trial, the necessity of taking steroids to return my liver to normal accelerated my cataract development and resulted in two surgeries within two months.

The weakness I experienced still makes me reluctant to walk in the neighborhood. I'm still battling back to a regular exercise routine. At this point, I'd settle for an irregular routine.

But I can't mourn forever. I am changing my focus from what happened in the past to what I can do now.

Yes, I lost physical wellness. But I've taken the first steps to do something about it. I signed up at my local recreation center and contacted a personal trainer to set up a weight training program.

Yes, I did a lot of stress eating and regained all the weight I lost and then some. I'm on a mission to get back to a healthy weight.

And yes, I lost any momentum in writing a new novel. The Lord directed me to a new project, which you now hold in your hand.

It's easy for us to focus on past failures and let them color our future. It doesn't have to be that way with physical problems. It works the same way with spiritual issues. We can be so focused on past failures we can't see anything else. We don't need to let the past determine the future.

A local remodeling company has a helpful slogan: "Take it like it is and make it what you want it." I can't change the past, but with God's help I can change my future.

"I will repay you for the years the locusts have eaten . . . and you will praise the name of the LORD your God who has worked wonders for you; never again will my people be shamed."
—Joel 2:25–26

43

TEAR DOWN THIS WALL

Blessed is he who expects nothing, for he shall never be disappointed.

—Alexander Pope

Watching cancer patients go through treatments is tough on the infusion nurses. They want to celebrate success, not worry the drugs they inflict will do more harm than good. It wrenched my own heart to see some patients' emaciated bodies hooked up to IV drips.

On my last day of treatment, my nurse handed me a Certificate of Completion, signed by the infusion center staff. She told me to ring the ship's bell fastened to the wall on my way out. That thing was loud! I heard a lot of shouts from the nurses celebrating the event. It reminded me of the scene in *It's a Wonderful Life* when the bell rings because an angel has gotten her wings. I should have been ecstatic. I wasn't.

I thought I'd be elated when the doctor finally told me, after two surgeries and three different treatments, that I was having my last infusion that day. I wasn't. Trying to force myself to grin or laugh did nothing because it didn't change how I felt inside.

It was weird. Everyone I told was thrilled. Why wasn't I?

A friend had important insights for me to consider. I'd been disappointed again and again. I thought the first surgery took care of the melanoma when the surgeon declared clear margins.

It didn't.

Then I was confident the second surgery would.

It didn't.

I was lured into a false sense of safety when the doctor wanted to treat me with immunotherapy "just to be on the safe side." The first two infusions lulled me into thinking I'd have no side effects. Just before my third one, a rash developed that was a harbinger of a horrible two months before recovery.

Then I entered a clinical trial in high hopes I would advance medicine while becoming cancer free. Nope.

When the doc explained he would be trying another drug on me, he touted his success using this particular immunotherapy. I was positive I would say, "Bye, bye, cancer," in short order. Instead, I ground out over a year of treatment without a clear end in sight.

Because of my up-and-down emotions, I had built up a wall around myself to prevent further dashed hopes. The problem was, when I really had good news, I couldn't grab hold of it because some part of me had built this wall—a wall that blocked me from joy as well as disappointment.

I learned, instead of grumbling about the part of me who had built it, I should instead acknowledge the protection that the overly enthusiastic guard inside me provided. I adopted a phrase used often toward military personnel: "Thank you for your service." I then gave it an honorable discharge, hoping it wouldn't reenlist. With God's help, the guards will leave and the wall will crumble.

I hope you or your loved one is at the end of successful treatment, but your emotions could be as confusing as mine. It's okay. Those protective walls were there for a reason. Now it's time for the fireworks and the dynamite.

Praise be to the L ORD my Rock, who trains my hands for war,
my fingers for battle.
—Psalm 144:1

44

REINVENTING MYSELF

He lifted me out of the slimy pit, out of the mud and mire; he set my feet on a rock and gave me a firm place to stand.

—Psalm 40:2

I felt rudderless after the doc decided he could discontinue my cancer treatments. *Who am I?*

My hubby had an insight that rang true: "Your identity has been wrapped up so long in being a cancer patient that, now that it's over, you've lost yourself." Bingo.

I needed to reinvent myself. I'd dropped most activities during my four-year battle. It was time to analyze what I wanted to do. I started doing fun stuff, with mixed results.

First, I pulled out a jigsaw puzzle, since I'd enjoyed building one at my sister's house when I visited. I wondered if it was a mistake considering we have two curious cats. I set it up on a card table and covered it carefully with a tablecloth when I wasn't working on it. However, one of said cats pulled the cloth off the puzzle, played with the pieces, and ruined a good chunk of my efforts. Scratch that idea.

I pulled out my long-neglected knitting to discover cat interference there as well. They never met a ball of yarn they couldn't turn into a tangled mess.

With extra time and more energy, I decided to do more cooking. Maybe I could discover a new entree my picky husband would enjoy with all of those new food magazine subscriptions. I had some successes but also ended up with a backlog of untried recipes. I wanted to keep up with all those magazines but found them languishing on my coffee table for weeks. I finally stopped renewing some of my subscriptions.

My next decision was to join a Bible study. I finally had time to do something that fed my soul. I looked forward to connecting with someone other than my nurses.

I decided to cut down on some of my social media. Although it's important for me to be engaged as a person and a writer, I discovered a lot of what I had been doing was, oddly enough, out of a feeling of obligation.

Although I dragged my feet on this next one, I started a blog about cancer. My posts feature innovative treatments and organizations that support patients. Except for an ongoing battle with my blog provider, I've enjoyed it.

I also decided to opt out of my volunteer museum work. After ten years, my position had been eliminated, and I had no desire to find a new one.

Then there was my writing. I decided to get serious about finishing this book. When I buckled down, I only needed to write seven more devotions to finish the first draft.

I joined a recreation center and spent three sessions with a personal trainer. Good start, but I haven't done a good job at following her fitness plan. I'm reluctant to make too many changes at once. No. To be honest, I'm lazy. Exercise sounds boring and too much like work.

In all of this, I needed to keep God in the loop. He knows my real self. He knows what I need to keep, what I need to drop, and what I need to pick up.

When you or your loved one has conquered cancer, it can feel overwhelming to pick up the pieces of the old life. Maybe that's not what you should do. Consider a new direction.

As I write this, the leaves are turning color. Fall will soon be here. The change of seasons reminds me my seasons change too. The season of cancer is over. Now is the time to establish new patterns and rhythms.

There is a time for everything, and a season for every activity under the heavens: a time to be born and a time to die, a time to plant and a time to uproot, a time to kill and a time to heal, a time to tear down and a time to build, a time to weep and a time to laugh, a time to mourn and a time to dance.
—Ecclesiastes 3:1-4

45

SCANXIETY

When I am afraid, I put my trust in you.

—Psalm 56:3

After four years of treatment, I was done with cancer. Or so I thought.

Sure, I would have CT scans every three months for two years, then less frequent ones. Big deal.

I didn't fool myself for long. The necessity of these scans unnerved me. The doc wanted to make sure the cancer hadn't returned. A wise precaution, but hardly comforting. That meant it *could* come back. Every scan before the tumors disappeared had spiked my fears the treatment would stop working. It happens. I dreaded the appointments with my oncologist to review the latest scan.

During a review of my first CT scan after stopping treatment, I expected my oncologist to say it showed no evidence of cancer. That's not what he told me. My scan revealed two enlarged lymph nodes under my right armpit. My *right* side, not the side where surgery had removed seven out of eleven lymph nodes. That scared me.

Although my doctor explained it could be the aftereffects of treatment, he wanted a biopsy to make sure. He assured me the procedure would use a tiny needle and I would be under sedation. I assumed that meant I wouldn't feel the pokes. Wrong. The nodes in question proved elusive and the surgeon had to poke me again and again. All that poking hurt when it happened and gave me a few days of discomfort as well. And of course, I worried that the result would show cancer regardless of the doc's reassurances.

In the meantime, my dentist noticed a lesion on my tongue. She wanted to wait three weeks to see if it would disappear.

It didn't.

She sent me to an oral surgeon who gave me a steroid rinse to use for two weeks. That should have taken care of it.

It didn't.

So I got a second biopsy five days later. That one was even more painful since the oral surgeon used bigger needles to puncture my tongue and to administer the numbing drug. The surgeon removed the lesion, which blissfully resulted in little pain afterward, but I was having more fun than humans are allowed.

To make things worse, the tissue from the tongue had to be sent to the University of Iowa for analysis, which meant a ten-day wait to hear the results. Also, I was reminded of a friend who'd had extensive surgery because of tongue cancer.

Now I was near panic. Had the cancer spread to previously unaffected areas? I couldn't go through more infusions again after being positive I was cancer free. I just couldn't.

I bit my nails until biopsy result number one came in from the lymph nodes. No cancer. Whew.

I waited another few days before results number two came from the University of Iowa. Inflammation of the tongue, no cancer.

The oncologist and oral surgeon agreed that those silly antibodies of mine were working overtime, like grave diggers who'd already exhumed a body but kept digging. The lymph nodes and tongue weren't the only things affected, however.

I developed patches of itchy eczema in various places. That nearly slammed me into PTSD as I remembered the good old days with the first immunotherapy and a resulting rash that kept me scratching day and night.

My skin, mostly on my arms, also became bleached in splotches. My oncologist commented on it. Apparently my ramped-up immune system couldn't distinguish between melanoma (the disease) and melanin (skin pigment). He said that was a good sign. I didn't believe him. What if those super antibodies decided my liver was tastier?

Hubby and I celebrated the biopsy results with dinner out. Christmas was coming, but we'd already received a wonderful present. However, I couldn't celebrate because worry still strangled me.

I needed to learn all over again God had things under control, regardless of biopsies. This will be a constant battle, since CT scans will be a regular part of my checkups. Will the next one show no cancer or reveal something suspicious? Will I need to suffer through more biopsies to discover the truth?

Can I really trust God?

I don't have a crystal ball, and God rarely tells me his plan. I can either chew my fingernails to stubs or rest in his peace.

I choose the latter.

Lord, trusting you when we're paralyzed by fear is beyond our capabilities. Help us to rest in your plan when we don't know the outcome. Amen.

46

SHE IS BRAVE

Reputation is an idle and most false imposition; oft got without merit and lost without deserving.

—Shakespeare, *Othello*

A popular bumper sticker reads, "Help me be the kind of person my dog thinks I am." For me it should read, "Lord, help me be the kind of person my *friends* think I am."

Many people tell me I'm so brave in my fight against cancer or I'm so strong in my faith. If they only knew the truth.

My reaction to the diagnosis of cancer wasn't just fright. It scared me out of my wits. The word *cancer* strikes fear in everyone who is diagnosed with it, as well as those who love them. However, thanks to advances in medicine, cancer is no longer a death sentence. Instead of a survival rate of six to nine months for patients with melanoma, doctors can estimate ten to twelve years of life with new drugs.

Survival rate: another term that frightens me. A survival rate of ten years means half the people who have the disease have died within ten years after diagnosis. It sounds a whole lot better than six to nine months, but I still don't like it.

There's no guarantee I'll be in the group that survives ten years or more. The uncertainty paralyzes me into thinking my life will be over in ten years and I might as well plan my funeral.

Death isn't something humans usually think about, but cancer patients like me think about it a lot. The Grim Reaper looming over us is enough to take the "brave" out of anyone.

Fear isn't anything new. Even heroes of the faith like Joshua were scared out of their sandals. So how did Joshua get past that? As I read about Joshua, I lost count of the number of times God told him directly or through others, "Do not fear; do not be discouraged."

Joshua's challenges aren't that different than ours. We aren't fighting actual armies, but we have cancer as an enemy. What's worse is our enemy is invisible unless it shows up in a CT scan.

So how do we become as courageous as our friends think we are?

We become brave by relying on the same friends who think we're brave. Confessing our fears somehow diminishes them because now they're in the open. And now those same friends become prayer warriors who fight the fear.

As we confess our fears to God, he gives us confidence and strength. This is not an instant solution but a learning process.

Reading about other people in the Bible who faced impossible odds and overcame them has encouraged me. In a devotional later in this book, I'll tell you what I learned from Jehoshaphat, Hezekiah, and Nehemiah.

I have a plaque on my desk that says, "She Is Brave." It's not a statement of what I am but what I can become with God's help.

Lord, we long to face cancer with bravery instead of fear. Help us to find our strength in you. Amen.

GOD'S WORD TO THE RESCUE

"Do not be afraid or discouraged because of this vast army. For the battle is not yours, but God's."

—2 Chronicles 20:15

Sometime after my second surgery, the oncologist wanted me to get an X-ray of my lungs and an MRI of my brain to make sure the melanoma hadn't spread.

If I hadn't been scared before, I was now. Melanoma likes to settle in the brain.

Around that time, I did a search of the times God said, "Do not fear; do not be discouraged." I can't list them all here. God told Joshua this so many times through so many people, I lost count.

Through this search, the stories of three men especially impacted me. These men faced certain annihilation but met the battle with prayer and with God's strength: Jehoshaphat, Hezekiah, and Nehemiah. They're great examples to me of how to fight and win, even against cancer.

Jehoshaphat, king of Judah, faced impending war with the Moabites, Ammonites, and Meunites, recorded in 2 Chronicles 20 When he learned a vast army was coming to attack Israel, the firs thing he did was pray. I wish I could say I did the same when I learned I had malignant melanoma, but I was too busy sobbing to form a coherent prayer.

Then Jehoshaphat ordered a choir to sing praises at the head of the Israelite army. Frankly, I would have declared a bad case of laryngitis before I'd get into that position. Risky business. What if God didn' come through?

The result of this man's faith? The Moabites and Ammonites slaughtered the Meunites, then turned and killed each other. All the Israelites had to do was collect the plunder.

In King Hezekiah's case, Sennacherib, king of Assyria, threatened Jerusalem with destruction, recorded in 2 Kings 19 and 2 Chronicles 32 The Assyrian army was camped outside the city gates. Hezekiah prayed. That night, an angel of the Lord killed 185,000 men in the Assyrian camp. Sennacherib withdrew in disgrace and was later assassinated.

My last example is Nehemiah, who returned from Babylonian captivity to rebuild the wall of Jerusalem. The story of his work is recorded in Nehemiah, chapters 2–6. The enemies of the Jews didn't like his plan one bit. They progressed from being disturbed to ridiculing to plotting all-out war. The Jews prayed for deliverance but also set a guard. Opposition tried to frighten and then to intimidate Nehemiah, but he wouldn't budge. Result: the wall was rebuilt, and the enemies realized it all had been done with the help of God.

We face enemies in the form of cancer, cancer treatments, grueling schedules of tests, infusions, and debilitating side effects. These opponents can overwhelm us, but we, like these biblical heroes, have an almighty and compassionate God on whom we can rely.

Lord, the cancer we face threatens to crush us like the armies of old. Help us to rely on your strength and not our own. Amen.

ACTION STEP:

Read the accounts of these three men.

4 8

CHOOSE JOY

Let us live while we live.

—Philip Doddridge

We have a choice in our cancer. We can either be miserable and make everyone else miserable, or we can reflect joy.

Now, I'm not minimizing the struggles you or your loved one go through in the journey toward a possible cure. Cancer is a scary diagnosis. Sometimes the treatment seems worse than the disease. And in this life, we have no guarantee we will be alive two years from now.

Two surgeries to remove tumors from my upper arm were painful. I'm not a fan of surgery since it invariably makes me vomit for a day. That's just the side effect from the anesthesia. The next problem is the aftermath of surgery. I'm a pain wimp. You know it's going to hurt when the doc prescribes super-duper-strong pain medication. I also have the dubious honor of having gotten stitches removed. Oh, and should I mention the long-term results of said surgery? I had a crater on my arm and decreased strength. I had to give up yoga for a while and ask surly supermarket baggers to haul my groceries.

And those side effects during treatment! Who can find joy in that?

I hope you or your loved one have experienced an easier road to a cure.

But in the middle of the battle with cancer, as in any other disaster in life, we can choose joy. It isn't fazed by the awful things we endure for the sake of treatment. It focuses on the positive things—sun on our faces, the antics of our cats, or even a good nap.

And guess what? A positive attitude can help our body to heal. When we're depressed, our attitude affects everything, including our antibodies. A happy T cell is an effective T cell.

I encourage you to look beyond your cancer. Don't let the disease overwhelm you, but overwhelm *it* instead.

I'm a big fan of the original *Star Trek* series. In one episode, an entity caused anger and infighting, even among the crew. The ultimate solution was laughter. The same principle applies to us.

So find a funny movie or an encouraging friend. Read a good book. Talk to that elderly and feisty neighbor. Join a cancer support group. Laughter may not cure the cancer, but it makes conquering it a whole lot more fun.

A friend offers this greeting on her voicemail: "Have a great day, because you know, we have that choice."

Choose joy.

My candle burns at both ends; It will not last the night; But ah, my foes, and oh my friends—It gives a lovely light!
—Edna St. Vincent Millay

ACTION STEP:
Invite some friends over for a board game.

49

IT'S MY PAIN

Each one should test their own actions. Then they can take pride in themselves alone, without comparing themselves to someone else, for each one should carry their own load.

—Galatians 6:4–5

In my cancer journey, I joined a writer's group for patients and care-givers my hospital sponsored. As I mentioned previously, I signed up with a self-serving desire to get feedback on the devotional I was writing (this one). I planned to encourage them with a deep spiritual message. At the very least, I expected a group that would improve my writing. I was wrong.

The class started with an assignment given at the first meeting, which I missed. The moderator didn't send me the instructions. (He had the wrong email address.) I showed up at the workshop with nothing to offer.

The rest of the members discounted their writing abilities, claiming they couldn't write. But as they read aloud their beautiful literary prose and poetry, I wondered why I was there. I doubted they'd relate to the humorous adventure I had with a radioactive tracer and my husband's Geiger counter, nor the spiritual applications I attempted to make.

I attended the second meeting with the same feelings. I was the odd person out with prose designed to evoke laughter and deep truth to ten people whom I doubted had strong faiths.

At this second meeting, however, I discovered the goal wasn't to teach writing. The workshop was a cathartic way for the participants to express the pain of their cancer journeys, which they did.

Again, I felt out of place. One participant struggled with brain cancer that caused seizures. One had Stage IV lung cancer, two had lost their husbands, and one woman was in palliative care because the doctors could do nothing more to stop or reverse her disease.

In listening to the others' stories, I started to discount my own. I'd had horrible side effects, but that was two years ago. My melanoma had metastasized but was successfully being treated with immunotherapy. I had high hopes I would soon be cancer free, unlike the experiences of others in the room.

Besides comparing myself with others in that workshop, I saw many patients in the blood center who arrived in wheelchairs and could hardly lift their heads. Someone I met in the infusion center was enduring yet another round of drugs administered over three hours. Mine was a quick half-hour, hardly enough time to read a few chapters from my latest escape novel.

So I became reluctant to share my own story and instead resorted to humorous anecdotes.

Then I realized I was avoiding the real issue: I had cancer and didn't want to face the feelings it evoked.

My struggle was real. I got fatigued after each treatment. I became weary of the rounds of blood draws, doctor's appointments, infusions, and occasional scans. Go to the hospital, take my medicine, repeat. As treatment continued after four years of surgeries, immunotherapy treatments, and side effects, I saw no relief. The doc showed me CT scans every three months that proved the treatment was kicking out the cancer. I just wanted it to be over. Those were *my* fears, *my* battle, and *my* pain.

I'm glad I'm now free from cancer, but anxiety about the future consumes me. Will I remain in remission, or will the cancer return? Will the drug still work the second time? Will I return to that treatment treadmill? I still have emotional pain.

A strange thing happened at this workshop. Instead of me inspiring these aspiring writers, they inspired me. They're persevering. They're expressing their own struggles.

With God's grace, I'll learn to express mine.

Lord, it's easy for us to compare ourselves with other cancer sufferers and discount our own pain. Help us to recognize and express our fears of the enemy we don't want to admit we have. Amen.

50

I WILL NOT BE SHAKEN

Truly my soul finds rest in God; my salvation comes from him. Truly he is my
rock and my salvation; he is my fortress, I will never be shaken.

—Psalm 62:1–2

I'd like to say I have an unshakable faith in God. I can't.

You or your loved one has experienced, like I have, the terror of cancer firsthand. Even if the treatment is working, even if the doc has declared us in remission, cancer free, cured, or whatever phrase he prefers, the niggling doubt remains. *He says he can't find the tumor, but am I really cured? What if the cancer comes back? What if it shows up somewhere else?* What if, what if, what if.

Cancer will always be the threat under our feet, waiting to turn into a 10.5 earthquake and bury us under the rubble. Sometimes I wonder if it would be better if the cancer returned. At least then, the monster would be out in the open and not a black cloud, impossible to grasp.

I can try to escape by employing my favorite avoidance tactics: bury myself in an overwhelming to-do list, bake banana bread until my husband's coworkers get tired of it (not likely), read sci-fi novels, watch movies. They don't change the situation or me.

Yes, there's no guarantee, with cancer or with life itself. As my husband likes to say, "Life can break at any seam." But God remains God, regardless of my lack of faith.

I think David, the author of the Psalms, knew fear. He wrote the above verse and so many others as if he was trying to convince himself that his faith was unshakable. It's a good verse to memorize.

Reciting a phrase of faith is not a cure-all for our lack of trust. It does, however, put us in a frame of mind in which God himself can speak into our fear and assure us of his strength.

One day in a mall, I passed a store that offered T-shirts with Christian slogans. The one that read "I will not be moved" caught my eye. I thought of getting that shirt. I couldn't do it. I don't feel that brave.

Fear is not something we can wish away or rebuke with an inspirational T-shirt. We can't fight it.

But God can.

> **We are hard pressed on every side, but not crushed; perplexed,
> but not in despair; persecuted, but not abandoned; struck
> down, but not destroyed.**
> **—2 Corinthians 4:8–9**

ACTION STEP:
Read Psalms 16, 30, 55, 62, and 112.

5 1

FEAR

How does one kill fear, I wonder? How do you shoot a spectre through the heart, slash off its spectral head, take it by its spectral throat?

—Joseph Conrad

f you aren't afraid in your journey through cancer, you haven't been paying attention.

I can't think of any other disease that strikes terror in one's heart more than cancer. Even though it's not a death sentence nowadays with the miraculous advances in medicine, "death sentence" is our first thought.

There are some scary diagnoses and prognoses out there. Some forms of cancer, such as pancreatic and esophageal cancer, are often discovered too late for effective treatment. Up until 2011, there were few options for melanoma treatment. And since melanoma likes the brain, I fear that one day it'll settle in and call mine home.

Side effects. I couldn't stand the thought of being sick. And unfortunately, the side effects I feared most came true: vomiting, diarrhea, fatigue, chemo brain.

Those side effects brought new fears. I was afraid to use the stair in our home. I had a heightened fear of falling. With every bite of food I took, I worried how sick it would make me. I even developed a dread of taking pills, including the one to help with nausea, because I gagged once.

And, of course, there's always fear of recurrence. *What if cancer shows in the next scan?* I dreaded getting the scans and especially meeting with my doc to discuss them.

What do we do with the fear? Some calming exercises can help, like walking and deep breathing. But emotional tricks don't touch the spiritual realm. The real issue lies with our perception of God.

Will I trust God for the outcome, whatever it is? Is he even trustworthy. Sometimes I wonder. Yet I'm convinced God is faithful. He has a track record, unlike the drug I took which is so new even oncologists can't predict its future. My trust must be in God and not in science or oncology.

I pray God will continue to grow my faith to echo the words of the psalmist:

God is our refuge and strength, an ever-present help in trouble. Therefore we will not fear, though the earth give way and the mountains fall into the heart of the sea.
—Psalm 46:1–2

SWING LOW, SWEET CHARIOT

When the perishable has been clothed with the imperishable, and the mortal with immortality, then the saying that is written will come true: "Death has been swallowed up in victory."

—1 Corinthians 15:54

Regardless of our stage of cancer, death has a habit of taunting us.

I've talked to some cancer patients who have a positive attitude they'll beat cancer. That's the hope of every one of us. But regardless of our faith or lack of it, regardless of the path this disease takes, death will eventually find us all.

The bigger question is what happens after cancer. Although our fight can consume us, this physical life is only a drop in the lake of eternity. God created us to live forever. Our hope must lie in God, not in the latest medical breakthroughs.

There's no guarantee I'll remain in remission. Although current survival rates for melanoma have increased from nine months to twelve years, thinking about it still scares me. The term "survival rate" means at one point on the life chart, half of the patients are still living. Of course that means half have died. So which camp am I in?

I struggle to keep the saying in mind, "I don't know what the future holds, but I know who holds the future." It's a nice saying, and a true one, but sometimes it feels like the well wishes I hear from acquaintances. I appreciate the sentiment; don't get me wrong. But if all I had to lean on was positive thinking, I would be lost. I'm not good at that kind of thing.

Lest you think I'm a religious nut, well, I am. That said, I struggle with end-of-life questions like everyone else. I wish I didn't have to have CT scans regularly because with each one, I fear it'll show the cancer has returned. But the bottom line is, I do know who holds the future.

The real trick in facing death is to know who's already faced it and conquered it.

As organs in the Body of Christ, as stones and pillars in the temple, we are assured of our eternal self-identity and shall live to remember the galaxies as an old tale.
—C. S. Lewis, *The Weight of Glory*

100 WORDS OF HOPE

I urge you today – whether you are the cancer patient or you are the caregiver – not to become a victim of cancer. Do not let this disease seem more powerful than it is. Do not let it *fill your mind, or destroy your hope.* It has no power to do those things unless you allow it to. As you take this unwanted journey with cancer, I believe you are going to discover two important, incredible, life-changing truths: *You are a lot stronger* than you think, and *God is a lot greater* than you think.

From Lynn Eib, *Fifty Days of Hope: Daily Inspiration for your Journey through Cancer* (2012), www. lynneib.com Used with permission.

RESOURCES

This is not an exhaustive list of all cancer organizations and support groups. I don't have enough space. This will give you some of the well-known as well as lesser-known foundations that raise funds, educate the cancer patient, and provide support. Being listed here does not imply I endorse these organizations.

American Cancer Society—Funds and conducts research, shares expert information, supports patients, and spreads the word about prevention. www.americancancersociety.org

American Cancer Society Cancer Action Network—Offers training to help cancer patients make their voices heard in the halls of government. Presses lawmakers and candidates to support laws and policies that strengthen the fight against cancer. www.fightcancer.org

CancerCare—Offers financial assistance and counseling, support groups, and patient education. Also provides free wigs and breast prostheses to women who have lost their hair or a breast as a result of cancer treatment. www.cancercare.org

Cancer Sucks—Raises funds for cancer research. Provides list of cancer organizations, hospitals, support groups. Sells T-shirts and other merchandise with "Cancer Sucks" logo. www.cancersucks.com

Cancer Support Group—This Facebook group is open to all that want to listen, read, learn, comment, and share their story or treatment their good news or the bad news. Started by Mark A. Sibley, MD

Center for Advancement in Cancer Education—Provides educa tional materials for cancer prevention and control, counseling for indi viduals battling cancer, training/certifications for doctors and othe health professionals, public seminars, and conferences. www.beat cancer.org

Eagle Mount—Organization in Bozeman, Montana, that helps chil dren with disabilities and cancer. Provides adventure programs fo children and young adults who have disabilities or who have cancer o are in remission. www.eaglemount.org

EBeauty Community—Accepts donations of used wigs, refurbishe them, and provides them free of cost for women going through cance treatment. www.ebeauty.com

Epic Experience—Offers adult cancer thrivers a free week-long outdoor adventure in the Colorado Rockies. www.epicexperience.org

First Descents—Provides outdoor adventures for young adults impacted by cancer and other serious health conditions. www.firstdes cents.org

Head Covers Unlimited—Sells head coverings in numerous styles www.headcovers.com

Hope Scarves—Shares scarves, stories, and hope with people facing cancer. Survivors can request a free scarf then return it with their story for the next woman. www.hopescarves.org

Live By Living—Connects cancer survivors and their caregivers with nature and one another. www.livebyliving.org

Living Beyond Breast Cancer—Offers to breast cancer patients resources that include publications, breast cancer hotline, conferences, interactive and online panel discussions, and webinars, plus additional services in the Greater Philadelphia Area. www.lbbc.org.

Look Good Feel Better—Teaches beauty techniques to people with cancer to help them manage the appearance-related side effects o cancer treatment. Program includes lessons on skin and nail care, cosmetics, wigs and turbans, accessories, and styling. www.lookgood-feelbetter.org

Lynn Eib: When God and Cancer Meet—Provides devotionals via email for cancer patients, list of Christian cancer support groups arranged by state, and devotional books available for sale. www.lynneib.com

Pancreatic Cancer Action Network—Provides patient services and advocacy, links to clinical trials, and a list of pancreatic specialists and centers; also sells "Wage Hope" apparel. www.pancan.org

Patient and Empowered—Blog by Christine Boyle, cancer survivor. www.patientandempowered.com

Sisters Network, Inc.—National African American breast cancer survivorship organization with affiliated chapters in several states. Organizes annual Stop the Silence 5K walk/run in the Houston area. www.sistersnetworkinc.org

Stand Up to Cancer (SU2C)— Matches cancer patients with clinical trials in their areas. www.standuptocancer.org

Stronghold Ministry—Website by Joe Fornear, cancer survivor. Provides free gift bags as encouragement to cancer patients, devotions via email, a Facebook prayer and support group (Stronghold Ministry Healing Prayer), and a weekly live Facebook prayer meeting. www.mystronghold.org

Susan G. Komen for the Cure (Susan G. Komen Breast Cancer Foundation)—Offers education online and holds conferences and 5K races throughout the nation. www5.komen.org

Wigs & Wishes By Martino Cartier—A network of salon owners, stylists, and beauty industry experts who provide women battling cancer with a wig at no cost, as well as granting wishes to children battling childhood cancer. www.wigsandwishes.org

ABOUT THE AUTHOR

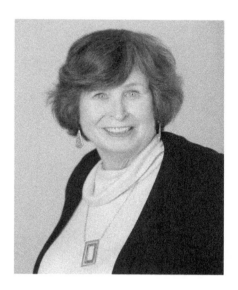

Bonnie Doran is a cancer survivor, a science fiction author, and contributor to numerous magazines. Her debut novel, *Dark Biology*, released in 2013. She lives in Denver, Colorado, with her husband of thirty-six years, John.

www.BonnieDoranBooks.com